It was not supposed to be this way Mum!

Helen Culliver

BSc, MSc, PhD, Dip Ed, Dip Pop Health

Disclaimer

This book includes sensitive information and discusses mental health issues in depth. It contains personal opinions and commentary regarding professionals, facilities and institutions in the mental health field. The content is based on the author's personal experiences and opinions. The views expressed are those of the author and do not necessarily reflect the opinions or experiences of others in relation to any professionals or organisations. Some names and places have been modified to protect the identity of individuals involved. The content may be distressing or triggering to some readers. Reader discretion is advised. If you are experiencing a mental health crisis, please seek help from a qualified professional.

Copyright © Helen Culliver 2025

All rights reserved.

This book is copyright. Apart from any fair dealing for the purposes of private study, research, criticism or review, as permitted under the Copyright Act, no part may be reproduced or transmitted by any process without written permission.

Inquiries should be addressed to:
Helen Culliver
penchantwriting@gmail.com

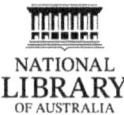 A catalogue record for this book is available from the National Library of Australia

It was not supposed to be this way Mum!

ISBN 978-1-7641553-0-4 (paperback)
ISBN 978-1-7641553-1-1 (ebook)

Cover Art by Alex Cameron
Cover Design by Clive Cameron

Contents

Acknowledgements v

Story players vii

Abbreviations xiii

Preface xv

Part 1 Alex's story 1

  Chapter 1 Childhood 3

  Chapter 2 Meeting the increased challenges 17

  Chapter 3 The good years 35

  Chapter 4 Misjudgement and overreaction 51

  Chapter 5 Doctors moved on, but Alex was stuck 77

  Chapter 6 Too hard so just increase restriction 97

  Chapter 7 Not wanted but not released 117

  Chapter 8 Indefinite incarceration 141

  Chapter 9 Despair then remarkable hope 171

  Chapter 10 Even if discharged, only by exile 195

  Chapter 11 Out of the frying pan.... 221

  Chapter 12 Too little, too late 249

  Chapter 13 The threat of homelessness 273

  Chapter 14 Inexorable decline 299

  Chapter 15 The end result 323

Part 2 The issues needing attention 353
1. The foremost issues 357
2. Auxiliary issues 381
3. Health's interface with community 395

Epilogue.. 409
Attachment - ASH1L de novo mutation 417

Acknowledgements

I would like to thank all those people who made an extraordinary effort to help Alex over the course of his life and who encouraged me to document his story as worthwhile for getting improvements in the way people with his problems are treated. I am retaining their anonymity but there were some wonderful individuals.

I thank my sons, Ewen, Donald and Clive Cameron for their support while I cared for Alex and have had my head down writing, and their forbearance with all the additional anxieties they have experienced within the family. My daughter-in-law gave valuable time on many occasions to be my moral support at meetings and in communications where I needed to keep pushing Alex's rights and needs.

Thank you to those who gave their information about what happened with Alex, to fill my knowledge gaps. These existed despite my contemporaneous notes taken at every meeting and from most phone conversations.

Dr Jennifer Torr and Professor Julian Trollor kindly supported me in reporting this as a case study in mental health care for those with cognitive problems as part of the new national effort to improve the health of those with an intellectual disability.

I am grateful for the advice given from health consumer advocates Russell McGowan, who advised about making sure there were policy messages linked to the story, and Janney Wale who cautioned me about my anger detracting from the messages. She pointed out the unclear areas in an early manuscript and encouraged me to give details of Alex's upbringing and pre-2017 life, so that the subsequent disasters could be understood better.

Alice Solomons gave me badly needed editorial advice to improve the readability of my crude text.

Extended family members have provided support and practical help throughout the ordeals. My brother-in-law Paul Henderson critically read my text, encouraging me to publish.

Story players

I have used job titles without names for most members of Alex's health and disability teams, even if more than one person occupied that position. A small number of real names are used with permission. There were two special people who worked closely with Alex for whom I have given pseudonyms rather than an impersonal job title, which seemed to better suit their relationships with him. For most of the doctors involved with Alex in the last few years of his life I have assigned a letter of the alphabet in order of appearance in the story. I have used this system so that the reader will know when a new doctor appears, not to expect the reader to get a full profile of each doctor. The job titles used are as follows:

Allied health manager

Manager of allied health personnel, clinicians undertaking work allied to medical care, such as psychologists, social workers and occupational therapists, often used as a spokesperson for a hospital with next of kin or guardian.

Art therapist

Allied health personnel offering art sessions as therapy.

Assistant Director of Nursing (ADON, Dhulwa)

This nursing position has overarching responsibility for the nursing teams and administration of the facility.

Behaviour Specialist

Qualified in psychology and/or occupational therapy, these private specialists are engaged by the patient, usually with funding from the National Disability Insurance Scheme (NDIS), to assess behaviours of concern, prepare a model of care for community living and oversee its implementation.

Case Manager

Often qualified nurses, a case manager can be assigned to a patient's clinical team in the local Mental Health Service for assistance with community care.

Chief Psychiatrist

This position is for an experienced psychiatrist employed by the state or territory government to take a leadership role for the profession of psychiatry practiced in their jurisdiction, to monitor operations under the relevant Mental Health Act and the rights of those being treated by psychiatrists.

Clinical Nurse Consultant (Dhulwa)

This position works under the ADON as an advanced registered nurse leading the nursing practice at Dhulwa.

Clinical Psychologist

A psychologist who applies their knowledge of complex human problems to the assessment and treatment (non-medicinal) for improved mental health of the patient.

Community Mental Health Service

Local community mental health services are given responsibility for the mental health needs of people living within a specified geographical area. The service includes a clinic for care of patients on clozapine, requiring monthly blood tests and a new prescription each month on a doctor's viewing of the blood results. If a patient changes address, they can come under a different service with different clinical staff.

Psychiatrist

A doctor qualified as a specialist practitioner capable of expert independent judgment in psychiatry.

Disability Support Worker

A certificated personal care worker who can be selected on the basis of a good personality fit and common interests with the client, and who will participate in client specific behaviour support training and model of care protocols. Good will and commonsense form part of a good worker in this field. They are employed in the private sector and not by the National Disability Insurance Agency (NDIA). They existed before the NDIS was created but numbers have increased since the introduction of the NDIS which has increased the availability of funding for this role.

Disability support worker provider (Support Worker organisation)

A private sector organisation which selects, trains and manages a team of disability care workers for a client. They are funded through the client's NDIS Plan but do not work for the NDIA. There can be several administrative positions within the organisation who liaise and get to know the client's case well.

Dual disability psychiatric expert

A psychiatrist with qualifications enabling expert dealing with psychiatric patients with a cognitive disability.

Guardian (now called Representative)

The person legally appointed by the ACT Civil and Administrative Tribunal (ACAT) under the *Guardianship and Management of Property Act 1991* to represent the affected person's interests in all matters including health. I, Alex's mother, was his guardian since he was 18 years old.

House manager/leader

This manager/coordinator works in the client's residence, getting to know the client, managing the worker team, trouble shooting and working with the resident's managers if these differ from the support worker organisation.

Occupational therapist

This allied health worker makes functional assessments of a patient including their capabilities to live independently. In hospitals they will introduce programs to assist the patient in recovery and prepare for community living.

Physiotherapist

This allied health worker helps a patient with mobility problems and suggests exercises for fitness and strength.

Public Advocate

The Public Advocate is an independent statutory authority funded by the state or territory government. They seek to protect the rights and interests of vulnerable people. The Office of the ACT Public Advocate was represented at multiple meetings and Tribunal hearings about Alex from 2017 to 2022.

National Disability Insurance Agency Planner

This position sits within NDIA. They take all the information about the NDIS participant for assessment and design of a funding package. They maintain contact with the participant's guardian/representative and support coordinator about the progress within NDIA for Plan approval and any additional information which might be required.

Neurologist

A specialist physician who deals with problems and diseases of the nervous system. They can be interested in brain disorders affecting behaviour but focus on motor and sensory functions. Alex saw a neurologist for his seizures.

Neuropsychiatrist

A Neuropsychiatrist is a specialist psychiatrist who tries to understand symptoms and attribute behaviour where psychiatry meets neurology. Neuropsychiatric disorders include schizophrenia, bipolar disorder and attention deficit hyperactivity disorder.

Social worker

The help from this position in hospitals included liaising with housing organisations, Government agencies such as Centrelink for pension payments, the judicial system as well as family.

Specialist Disability Accommodation Providers

These are property developers interested in the residential needs of those with selected disabilities. They take up the SDA funding from the NDIA for building special accommodation according to strict specifications in a range of categories. It is a difficult area of property development, sensitive to land availability and zoning, and considerations beyond usual residential development. Support from local government is essential. SDA is intended for only a subset of NDIS participants.

Support Coordinator

This person is very important for NDIS participants with complex needs. It is a private sector function funded by the participant's NDIS Plan. The support coordinator advises on Plan use and oversees the search for providers to be employed using the Plan funds. They can be pivotal in the search for accommodation and in how to approach the NDIA for review of funding and making applications such as for SDA. They can coordinate community team meetings for united action among different providers and liaise with the health sector and guardian. Alex had an ACT support coordinator and a Victorian support coordinator with both contributing for an overlapping period.

Abbreviations

ACAT	ACT Civil and Administrative Tribunal (for decisions under different Acts such as the *Mental Health Act 2015* and the *Guardianship and Management of Property Act 1991*)
ACT	Australian Capital Territory
ADON	Assistant Director of Nursing
AHCR	After Hours Crisis Response
AMHU	Adult Mental Health Unit (Canberra Hospital)
CATT	Crisis and Assessment Treatment Team
CIT	Canberra Institute of Technology
CNC	Clinical Nurse Consultant
COVID-19	Coronavirus disease 2019
DASA	Dynamic Appraisal of Situational Aggression
DFFH	Department of Families, Fairness and Housing (Victoria)
DMHU	Dhulwa Mental Health Unit
DSA	Disability Services Australia
GP	General Practitioner
EEG	electroencephalogram
HDU	High Dependency Unit (AMHU Canberra Hospital)

ICP	Individual Care Plan
ICU	Intensive Care Unit
ISRP	Integrated Service Response Program in the ACT Office for Disability
IST	Intensive Support Team (of DFFH)
IV	Intravenous administration
LDU	Low Dependency Unit (AMHU Canberra Hospital)
MACNI	Multiple and Complex Needs Initiative (Victoria)
MARG	Multi-agency Response Guideline
NDIA	National Disability Insurance Agency
NDIS	National Disability Insurance Scheme
NMS	Neuroleptic (i.e. antipsychotic) Malignant Syndrome
OCD	Obsessive Compulsive Disorder
OT	Occupational Therapist
PRN	pro re nata – for medication required as circumstances arise
PTO	Psychiatric Treatment Order
SDA	Specialist Disability Accommodation
SIL	Supported Independent Living

Preface

I wrote this book so that my son Alex's story is not lost as just another unfortunate but unfathomable life. This is a record of what happens when a case can be classified as "complex" while not taking full account of history and symptoms. His story is of professionals who operate with narrow thinking or closure to new thinking. Such short-sightedness is strange for professionals in emerging fields of neurodevelopment, neurodiversity and neurodegenerative conditions. His story reveals the lack of listening from doctors to either the patient or his guardians and carers, and lack of communication from doctors on what their rationales for treatments are. There were also people just not doing their jobs and poor systems within which to work.

I hope my insight into Alex's experience of a lack of proper care will raise awareness among fellow parents and interested professionals. Parents and carers need access to this sort of documentation of cases of paired disability: cognitive and psychiatric. I hope that it can encourage other parents to question and advocate for patients' rights. Health and disability professionals need to hear this story in order to learn what not to do and what should be done better in health and disability systems, separately and together.

Administrations, systems and ministers of government do not appear in good light in this drama. This book is a cry for recognition of human rights and avoidance of blaming the person with disabilities. Alex's tormented existence in his last years of life should be made explicit to society in order to do the right thing by his memory, at risk of suffering in vain, and to try to help others at risk of similar treatment.

This story is about more than Dhulwa Forensic Mental Health Unit ACT where Alex spent over three years. Following mainly workplace safety complaints, Barbara Deegan Chairperson of the Inquiry probed a range of issues and made her Final Report on 11 November 2022[1] making 25 recommendations. I understand Dhulwa has already learnt some hard lessons (some from Alex) and has been making an effort to improve from even before the Inquiry. Alex's full story can reinforce the findings of this Inquiry but it can go further. It can give the other dimensions to mental illness, giving context and meaning to the life Alex led. It highlights the bias in assessment and diagnosis when a patient has cognitive disability which was beyond the scope of the Inquiry. It adds grist to the findings of the Royal Commission into Violence, Abuse, Neglect and Exploitation of People with Disability (September, 2023) about the health service improvements required in general.

Finally, this book is an opportunity to tell Alex's story from the inside. While others have told their versions of Alex, either fired with rage (Small Town, Victoria) or to engage in patient blaming with release of his personal health information (his

---

[1]

https://www.cmtedd.act.gov.au/__data/assets/pdf_file/0003/2117271/Final-report-Inquiry-into-the-Legislative,-Workplace-Governance-and-Clinical-Frameworks-of-Dhulwa-Secure-Mental-Health-Unit.PDF

Dhulwa nurses), I think it important for Alex to have his own say through me. I used his owns words where I could, including for the title.

I have biological science qualifications which has affected the way I tried to understand Alex and to keep thinking of how he could best be helped throughout his life when no one else could. This book presents the story as far as I know it and I acknowledge that I do not have complete evidence. So much was hidden or kept from me. I believe Alex's death was premature and contributary factors were preventable. There are strong links between the poor health treatment he received and his last five years of decline and demise. I wrote this book very much as a mother wanting to do the very best for her son.

Part 1 Alex's story

Chapter 1 Childhood
1982 - 1994

Alex was born in 1982, our much wanted first born. It was an uncomplicated pregnancy and labour. I thought he was adorable and loved him very much. I found difficulties, however, from the first day, such as with feeding and settling. I did not expect all to be easy as a first-time mum. I worked through the issues so that he thrived regardless. It was only when my three other sons showed no such problems as new born babies, did I realise Alex's babyhood was an unusual challenge.

Another mother whose baby about the same age was cared for with Alex at a Family Day Care home remarked one day that Alex should be doing the same things as her daughter. This was not helpful. I tried to relax about milestones as I knew that the normal range could be wide. Alex began walking within the normal age range, but talking was more delayed, especially with appropriate story sequencing. While his cranial fontanelles closed early, his head grew at a normal rate.

I breast fed him until he was about 15 months old, using expressed milk when he was in care. He had some milk supplementation earlier when medical check-ups about poor weight gain scared me. He began solids from about 6 months.

Despite early poor weight gain he caught up after a few months. By the time he was ten, his weight was at the 90th percentile and his height above the 97th percentile.

From about 9 months, with teething, he suffered from several bouts of tonsillitis. He was often on antibiotics, if not for tonsillitis, for ear infections. With doctor's checks, some developmental delay was identified by age two. He was given an early pre-school place and was lucky enough to have a specially trained teacher who had many consultations with me about Alex's troubles. She was thinking ahead for schooling too, wondering whether he needed a special school. He was enrolled in physiotherapy sessions for a while to try to improve balance and coordination in 1987 (aged 5) and he was given exercises for general sensory motor function.

An occupational therapy assessment in that year concluded he was functioning to age in his manipulative skills, but his flow of movement, particularly with bilateral tasks was poor. He appeared to have a delay in fine motor writing and a program was recommended.

He did not attend a special primary school, but went to a mainstream school where a wonderful teacher in grade one taught him to read and write. His anxieties and social difficulties remained, leading to being easily upset at school and vulnerability to teasing. We moved his school for grade three (1991) because his first school was threatened with closure under ACT government rationalisation. The second school was a mistake lasting only six months, after which we moved to another local primary school which had the benefits of the best teachers from a previous school merger. He finished primary school there. He was able to have additional support in the classroom which he objected to at times, saying, "it makes me feel like a nut".

Alex was good at playing quietly by himself. He loved building blocks and Matchbox cars which he would line up carefully along ledges and shelves. His father made Alex a wooden two story garage with the upper floor for parking, which gave him hours of fun. He loved puzzles and being read to, especially if I used funny voices. He developed a love of movies and I admit I used *Mary Poppins* on VHS tape as a babysitter often.

Professional advice sought

In 1989, we took him to see a Sydney based neurologist after the grade one teacher observed *deja vu* episodes with Alex. He seemed to be having gaps in his awareness of place and time. She reported on one occasion he came back into the classroom after playtime saying "I think I have been here before". The neurologist could not detect anything on their examination to support epilepsy. He noted we, the family, might need help with his emotional and behavioural management. Where else could we look for help?

The approach from doctors was that the cause of his problems and the exact diagnosis would be impossible to uncover, so the best advice had to be about coping as parents. Alex needed special parenting for which we would need special skills. He developed fixations and persistence of tantrums. He was accident prone at home. A child psychiatrist, from whom we sought help with his behavioural issues in 1990, interviewed Alex on his own, possibly with an intention to question him about home life. It was as if without a medical diagnosis they entertained the idea there was damage in his upbringing. Internal Health letters expressed disappointment that I did not want to avail myself of further useful psychological help while I was adamant that Alex had a physiological source of his difficulties.

Also in 1989, a clinical neuropsychologist found Alex's intellectual performance in the upper end of the Low Average range but thought he was perhaps unwell with a respiratory infection that day and recommended further testing in a year.

1991 was a busy year following up possible diagnoses as well as shifting school. The child psychiatrist described Alex as a diagnostic dilemma but prescribed him thioridazine (50 mg at night), a first-generation antipsychotic. I had reported Alex being afraid of voices as if someone was in his room. The psychiatrist documented that he had not seen any psychotic symptoms in Alex but noted that Alex was more cooperative and less aggressive while being treated with this antipsychotic medication. He intended to discontinue this medication after a few weeks and rely on a psychologist to coach Alex out of his worries and outbursts. He described Alex as a nervous talkative boy who has mannerisms of the arms and face, which drew attention to himself and made it hard to make friends with other children. There was no diagnosis.

Space was made available also with a visiting Sydney psychiatrist who was very interested in interviewing us, as parents, as well as seeing Alex. He asked probing questions as if trying to psychoanalyse us and our relationship, but he suddenly refused to include Alex's case in his limited time in Canberra after only about three consultations.

Search for help widened

In 1991 I wrote a long list of concerns to be able to hand to doctors. I recorded that Alex was hardly ever still with movements including hand shaking, extraneous jaw movements, bouncing and whole body shaking. He would hum to himself and rush about. Alex began bizarre behaviours such as stuffing his mouth with tissues because it was "wet". He would use self-harm in scratching and hitting the sides of his head.

One of his obsessions at this time was avoidance of his younger brother Ewen (b.1985). Alex would not stay in the same room as Ewen. He would often gulp his meal so he could retreat to his own room quickly. When younger, the two boys had learnt to play with each other quite well even if Alex had to learn new controls to share and pair in games. Alex apparently began avoiding others at school at this stage, instead isolating himself mumbling.

Alex was convinced that boys at school hated him. He was preoccupied with being teased. I recorded my thoughts based on teachers' reports that perhaps he was making assumptions relating to old events or had an exaggerated idea of the harmful intent of others. I thought that the thioridazine had improved this behaviour which could have been interpreted as paranoia, but this was not conclusive. He took thioridazine for two years until October 1993.

Alex had poor self-esteem, telling me "I wasn't born to be happy", "I can't help being born with a head like this", "I wish I had never been born", "You should not have got the family together", "I told the kids at school I'd kill myself". He did not like his school photos and damaged them before bringing them home.

Alex's other brothers, Donald and Clive, were born in 1990 and 1993 respectively. Alex was always intrigued by the arrival of a baby and was very good with them initially. As they matured, he found it difficult to cope with any emotional friction.

In September 1991 I made contact with a Norwegian researcher interested in possible connections between absorbed peptides and neurological conditions such as autism. His articles interested me since Alex's doctors had not found a possible cause for his difficulties. The researcher was very helpful, and sent me instructions for processing two 24-hour urine samples from Alex which I posted for his research laboratory to analyse. From my processing of the samples, the researcher found residue spectra consistent with his surveys, for attention deficit disorder with hyperactivity, depression and hyperkinesia, with some psychotic features and a strong peak for aggression. He recommended a milk-free diet. This was all interesting but overall, we were not closer to a satisfactory diagnosis. We had tried a gluten-free and milk-free diet for a while without being convinced.

Through a paediatrician at Royal Canberra Hospital, we sought help with Alex's allergies concurrent with his frequent infections, nose and sinus issues. His frequent nose blowing needed to be checked for a physiological cause as well as his purported need to seek attention. The idea that food colourings could affect behaviour of children was also popular at that time. The skin-prick tests were done by a specialist in Sydney. According to the tests, Alex was very allergic to some moulds and environmental particles such as from dust and rye grass. He was allergic to some foods, to tomatoes for example and oddly, to rice, which is usually seen as benign with respect to allergenic properties. I remember that we had decided that an elimination diet would be too difficult at that stage given Alex's other issues, but I tried to minimise offenders.

I remembered that the pre-school teacher said that Alex behaved as if he was stimulus-deprived, which we both knew was not the case. In 1993 I sought help from a private organisation based in Sydney which offered advice and avenues for therapy for children with learning difficulties. She put me in touch with a Canberra based therapist who took Alex through a program intended to re-awaken responses to stimuli that normally start from birth. There was a name for his apparent difficulty – sensory integration dysfunction. Alex quite enjoyed this program and remembered the therapist fondly for the rest of his life. It was difficult to measure what help it was.

I spent his growing years trying to get help for him going from one specialist to another, acting as his case manager. The ACT Health service provided a case manager for short bursts but it was always unable to sustain such help due to lack of funding. No specialist wanted to know him, could not own him in their field as having a particular diagnosis, and told me they could not help. My records of his odd or worrying behaviours were consistent over a long period of time. He could be a dear, gentle child who could also be overwhelmed by life, manifesting in tantrums and family disruptive behaviours. I kept searching except for a brief period when I was worried about any negative effects of him hearing the persistent message that there was something wrong with him.

For example, I made an extensive record in December 1993 (11 years old) of his behaviours, likes and dislikes. This might be of interest for reflection on the phenotype Alex presented, as an idiosyncratic and enigmatic profile of behaviours among those with neurological disabilities.

Category	Description
Hearing things	Always hearing "annoying noises". He described these as air noises or people whispering. He showed sensitivity to distant quiet noises too.
Itches	He felt itchy all over. He obtained relief by licking fingers and wiping these on the affected parts. He often rubbed his knuckles into and around his eyes because they were itchy.
Nose congestion	Frequent blowing, often hard and noisily and always more frequently and strongly if agitated.
Causes of agitation	His brothers, crowds, not being understood when speaking, not being able to control games and activities with other children.
Habits (hyperactivity or mania)	Speech rapid and prolonged, rapid eating and resistance to food requiring chewing, preference for standing not sitting, tidying rituals, and wiping hands on the carpet.

Distress expression	Wailing without tears, slapping face until cheeks and lips bled, head hitting on the wall or desk and floor stomping.
Sleeping	He was hard to settle and then tended to be hard to wake in the morning. Frequent nightmares but these reduced compared to early childhood. He would position himself huddled on two pillows with occasional stretching out during the night.
Education to grade 5 at this stage	Average progress. Average to better in reading. Below average and variable in mathematics. The mechanics of writing was hampered by poor coordination. His expression suffered from lack of structure, poor sequencing, too many words, somewhat mimicking his speech problems. His art was naïve but had character.
Social skills	He got on well with adults with whom he was good at starting conversations. He would remember names and having met various people, for example on holidays. He did not make friends with peers well. He had immature preferences for games. At school he was liked and accepted by most of his classmates but was susceptible to some teasing from those outside his class. He was polite and aware his habits could be

	embarrassing. He coped well on school excursions.
Assessments	Paediatric, physiotherapy, occupational therapy, speech, psychology, neuropsychology, neurology, psychiatry
Likes	Odd noises which he would mimic and repeat. Playing short bursts of Michael Jackson, recording favourite other noises. Watching television alone crouched on the floor near the set. Listening to stories read to him Talking to Mum and being held by Mum Visiting people's homes and exploring. Lollies, cakes, whipped cream and ice-cream. Having space to himself. Gifts. Investigating by touching objects Walking. Early on, construction toys with blocks etc. Wearing shorts under long pants
Dislikes	Touch by most people. Annoying Noises. Staying at home Being in same room as brothers Loose clothing Clothing he finds itchy

A sort of diagnosis

By this stage we had accumulated a list of diseases and conditions which could be somewhat matched with Alex, from my reading and doctors' comments. He had bits of attention deficit disorder, Tourette's syndrome, obsessive compulsive disorder, hyperactivity, psychotic symptoms, possibly autism, and all with a query on a genetic basis. There was no environmental cause identified. There was no real help in the ACT.

It was the Chief Psychiatrist at the Children's Hospital in Sydney, who finally recognised that Alex "might be a bit sick" in 1993 (Grade 5, Alex eleven years old). In August 1994, this doctor wrote:

> Alexander suffers from a psychotic disorder of childhood which is as yet unspecified. He requires substantial anti-psychotic medication and has impairment of attention, concentration and on task behaviour with unusual behaviours and rushes of emotion over which he has very limited control. Despite this, his intellect is very much within the normal range and he is burdened by an insight into his own condition. He is one of the most impaired children with a normal intellect and within a caring family context that I know.

The doctor's description is consistent with later life descriptions for Alex when he was not on adequate medication. Noteworthy is the emphasis of this senior psychiatrist at this time on mental illness, not on intellectual disability. The main changes observed with Alex as he got older were the extremes of his "rushes of emotions" and changes related to intellect, which seemed to be diminishing with age. The intelligence testing was intermittent, however, and his grade 6 assessment (1994) was thought to be an underestimate because of his "medical conditions" by the school counsellor when the IQ scores were lower than as measured in 1989.

Even if it were an accurate observation that Alex's cognitive abilities declined with age, this could not have reduced his mental illness tendencies concomitantly. Any later demonstrations or evidence of poor cognition should not have discounted the likelihood that he had mental illness, even if that mental illness profile were not typical.

Despite the concerns of his pre-school teacher, Alex had learned to read and write and was very determined to try to keep learning, to be good and to do what was asked of him. Throughout his life I kept telling him he had abilities and that we appreciated his talents in art and craft, his roles in making family occasions joyous, especially at Christmas, and his energies in following multiple interests. I was determined that he have as many opportunities as possible to use his abilities.

While in The Children's Hospital Sydney Alex's drawing of Ronald MacDonald House in Camperdown won first prize to be used on the cover of their Annual Report 1994.

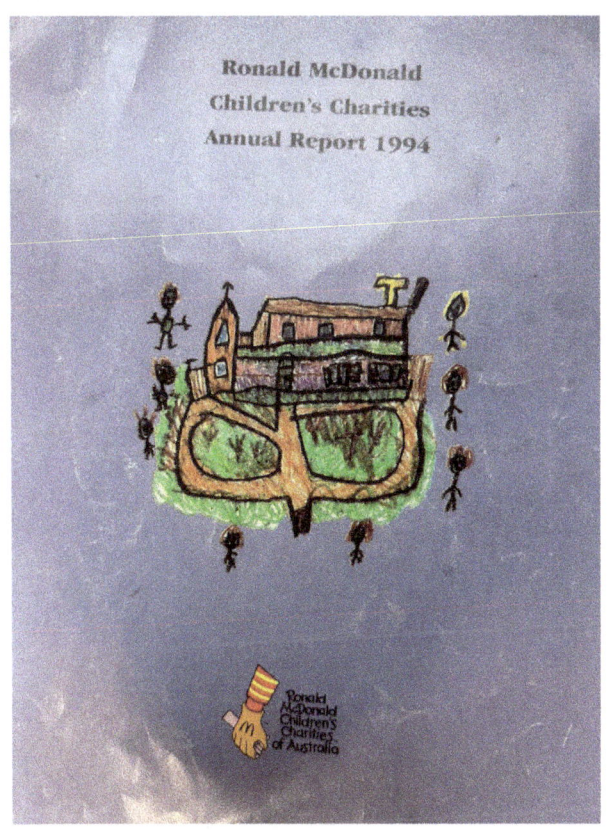

Whatever was his neurological issues, I believed that family love, provision of opportunities, support for his ideas and encouragement to participate would allow him to have a good life.

Chapter 2 Meeting the increased challenges
1995 - 2007

Alex's teenage years brought additional and more serious challenges, new psychiatric treatments and recommendations for a move away from mainstream schools. He lived at home which was always challenging for parenting and for his brothers now developing expressions of their frustrations. We did manage holidays at the beach or to Melbourne to see relatives. Occasionally we secured respite care for Alex but he was not enthusiastic about it.

He developed new or more extreme forms of his odd behaviours. His toileting became unmanageable. He would spend one or more hours there at a single visit, making it impossible to run the house to a timetable. He could use so much toilet paper that we frequently required a plumber. He fussed over house security and became excessively protective of his room and possessions. He would wear the same clothes until pressured into changing them. He did not want his soiled clothes taken to the laundry. He became anxious about school bus travel even though we were able to verify that there was no teasing or taunting – at least not routinely.

We commenced Alex in a Catholic high school for grade 7 where funding was found for an aide to help him adjust to the changes from primary school. We had investigated the local public high school where a wide range of intellectually disabled children attended. We did not think that Alex would cope with the environment there, especially with those children who were non-verbal or withdrawn in a corner.

I consulted a private clinical neuropsychologist in 1996. This professional was provided with the accumulated professional and school reports on Alex and a copy of his first EEG output. He said that all Alex's symptoms were suggestive of some episodic dysregulation syndrome. His symptoms seemed to have a similar underlying neurological/biochemical basis, resulting in problems in his ability to 'self-regulate' a whole host of physiological and psychological functions. Interestingly he thought Alex's hearing of voices were probably more in line with obsessive compulsive behaviour than with hallucinations. The clinical neuropsychologist was getting closer to the idea that there was a unifying explanation for all Alex's symptoms rather than seeing him as a collection of unrelated syndromes or strict division of cognitive disability from mental illness.

I kept using phrases such as "it is all neurological" regardless of how they tried to match a set of symptoms to a disease label.

We took Alex several times to the hospital Emergency Department from 1995 to 1998 briefly itemised as follows.

Year	Reason for visit	Doctor Comments
1995 12 years	Punched his father, kicked glass door: reported feeling frustrated that his mother was attending to the younger boys not him.	No clear diagnosis. Current medication haloperidol (antipsychotic) 5 mg at night, sertraline (antidepressant) 25g/day. Action: stop sertraline, give diazepam (sedative) as needed 5 mg, referral to Child and Adolescent Unit.
1996 13 years	Mother feels no one is helping and she is worried about the safety of the other children with his impulsiveness and irrationality.	Wait for referral to the Child and Adolescent Unit and meanwhile continue with the new child psychiatrist (who also soon moved away from Canberra), and the Chief Psychiatrist at the Children's Hospital in Sydney.
1997 14 years	Alex angry over a minor matter regarded as important to him. Assault of parents.	Alex to remain on haloperidol, 5 mg in morning, 3 mg at night. Description by doctor of Alex included drooped posture, rocking movements, straightening of sheet on trolley, fingering of water bottle. Rapid breathing, tic-like movements of the mouth.

		Not hallucinating. Alex reported he had difficulties with others and was worried about the future if there was not better medicine.
July 1997	Psychiatrist request to change medication under supervision	Medication changed from haloperidol to olanzapine (another antipsychotic) 5 mg at night after first reducing only evening dose of haloperidol. Diagnosis given as schizo-affective disorder.
April 1998 15 years	Brought by ambulance from airport where he froze in a foetal position after disembarking, refusing to go with his father who was there to collect him after his short holiday in Melbourne.	Mother arriving reduced his stress. Doctor noted medication risperidone (another antipsychotic) 3 mg twice daily and clomipramine (another antidepressant) 25 mg at night. Increased clomipramine to 125 mg for two days, then 150 mg nocte.
June 1998 15 years	Bizarre risky behaviours: face in very hot water to change his colour, face under tap water for half an	Presented very disturbed, protective movements to avoid touch, incoherent speech. Apart from recommendations that the face be kept clean to avoid infection, there was

	hour and constant rubbing of the face	nothing forthcoming on Alex's psychiatric state except a possibility he could be admitted to the private psychiatric hospital Hyson Green.

The family was very concerned and frustrated that there was no confirmed diagnosis and no help seemed possible. We kept managing as best we could. Alex's brothers had grown up with his quirks and outbursts but it was getting harder for them. After these years of trying to handle increasing troubles at school and call-outs to the Crisis Team (CATT) from home, something new was required.

New approach

I was pleased when Alex was seen by a new psychiatrist at the Child and Adolescent Unit who worked with the Chief Psychiatrist at Westmead. They decided in 1998 that Alex would benefit from being taken off his current medication and re-assessed in a secure facility which would allow for a possible replacement medication, clozapine, to be introduced under supervision. Alex was admitted to Redbank House in Sydney. This facility was very thorough in its assessments and very caring.

The consultant psychiatrist at Redbank House noted that Alex's treatment to date had resulted in only marginal improvements. He noted that the antipsychotics tried in series in recent times: risperidone (up to 9 mg daily), olanzapine (5 mg nocte) and most recently a return to haloperidol (5 mg twice daily) were not effective. The antidepressants clomipramine and citalopram were not effective for his obsessive-compulsive disorder nor for his anxieties. Sertraline (brand name Zoloft) was associated with new bizarre behaviours. The other antidepressants were not associated with adverse effects but were given at times when there were other behaviours which might have masked any similar effects to those of sertraline.

The clinical neuropsychologist at Redbank House performed a detailed assessment in August 1998. She reported he was very anxious at the testing. I have no record of what medication, if any, he was taking at this stage in his admission. Apparently, he tired easily while completing verbal tasks. The neuropsychologist concluded that at age 16 he could be characterised as mildly intellectually disabled. She made recommendations for a review of his schooling and for discipline about toileting.

We were able to make improvements in medication and schooling which meant improvements in Alex's way of life. Alex commenced clozapine which is an atypical antipsychotic usually given to those not responding to other antipsychotics. He was also prescribed the antiepileptic and calming valproate while he was still exhibiting severe head banging and tantrums. He was much calmer by March 1999. I have no record of the length of time he was taking valproate at this stage.

Alex attended a special school called Koomarri School in the ACT, with a later change of name to Black Mountain School, from the end of year 10 (1999) to age 20 years (2002). The teachers and the school organisation were fantastic. He adjusted and enjoyed his time there with its shift to education for life skills in hygiene, shopping and banking, work etiquette and crafts such as silk printing. They had great success in reducing the toileting issues. He was valued, gaining an award one year for his helping of others such as those in wheelchairs.

The psychiatrist from the ACT Child and Adolescent Unit moved to private practice so we followed him there to give continuity for Alex. We managed the clozapine monthly checks for agranulocytosis (loss of white blood cells) and renewed prescriptions with a workable crossover between public and private systems. Alex was tolerating clozapine well. He did not display the listed side-effects except sedation and hypersalivation. I have no record of the dosage. The hypersalivation on its own could be inconvenient but when responsible for aspiration pneumonia it was a serious side effect.

His better behaviour was due to his better medication as well as to the skills of his new school. It was evident that clozapine was the best medication tried to date. It was also emerging that clozapine on its own was insufficient as Alex was not symptom free and needed ongoing monitoring. I will give details here of Alex's medication refinements at this stage as it contributes to his profile of complexity to diagnose and treat.

The Chief Psychiatrist at the Sydney Children's Hospital and the Canberra Child and Adolescent psychiatrist had also decided to commence Alex on 5-hydroxytryptophan (serotonin precursor) to boost serotonin at synapses, given that the serotonin re-uptake inhibitors were ineffective. This was initially arranged through Westmead as an individual supply, as it was not registered on the Australian Register of Therapeutic Goods. When this supply ran out in 2001, I applied to the Therapeutic Goods Administration to make a personal importation on the basis of its effectiveness in Alex. We were able to maintain supply for a few years. Interestingly we did not observe any bizarre behaviours that might have been expected if it resulted in the same side-effect as from serotonin re-uptake inhibitors (e.g. sertraline, citalopram, clomipramine) occurred.

Alex was also prescribed aripiprazole (15 mg daily) with an explanation given to me that Alex's schizophrenia, if that is what he had, was not typical and warranted an additional attack. Aripiprazole has partial agonist (stimulant) [2] activity at dopamine and serotonin receptors which might benefit Alex, according to the Canberra Child and Adolescent psychiatrist. Manic symptoms were not mentioned as far as I remember. This psychiatrist foresaw that Alex's multiple problems could have arisen from closeness of different functional areas morphologically in the brain, in which the putative damage was non-discriminatory regarding function.

My records of Alex's psychiatric treatments have significant gaps for the next few years. The Child and Adolescent

---

[2]It is not known how agonist or receptor stimulation works against some aspects of psychotic symptoms. In comparison clozapine acts primarily as an antagonist at dopamine and serotonin receptors. Not enough is known about how these antipsychotics work as they do more than one thing in the nervous system anyway and there are subtypes of receptors favoured by a particular antipsychotic.

psychiatrist in private practice wrote notes at every consultation but refused to share these notes when later it was obvious that this would be very helpful. When Alex was in a public hospital or seen by public system psychiatrists, doctors being able to see a complete record was all important. I was naïve in thinking there was no need for me to keep parallel notes for the private consultations. In any case, Alex was relatively stable at that time. I tried writing to the private psychiatrist in 2014 to ask about his records of Alex taking sertraline because the Clozapine Clinic doctor was contemplating prescription of it again for Alex's obsessive compulsive disorder. I received no reply. Alex might have had a period in which valproate was removed from his regimen in the years prior to 2007.

Significant side effects emerging

Alex experienced a bout of pneumonia in 1999, thought to be possibly aspiration pneumonia as a result of the hypersalivation induced by clozapine. His X-ray showed opacity in the lower segment of his upper right lobe. He was treated with clindamycin. This was the first of several bouts of pneumonia. There was precedence for aspiration pneumonia among clozapine users [*Aspiration pneumonia possibly secondary to clozapine-induced sialorrhea* Hinkes R, Quesada TV, Currier MB et al., Journal of Clinical Psychopharmacology 1996, 16(6): 462-463.].

He went to the Emergency Department again in April 2001 because of chest pain on top of a urinary tract infection. The hospital discounted pneumonia and heart problems. His ankles were showing signs of swelling easily at this stage too.

While our main concerns were always about his psychiatric state, any physical and dental problems needed to be also tracked. Overall, his physical health seemed good and he seemed very strong and robust. His better behaviour enabled him to keep active and keep fit. We were optimistic about his future. I was able to give more time to the other boys.

Dental work required

It is worth describing at this point the dental orthodontic work and surgery that Alex had from 1992 to 2002 because the jaw growth that required rectification could have been related to the genetic abnormality eventually found in 2020. In 1992 an orthodontist took a head x-ray and reported:

> a tendency for backward positioning of the upper jaw relative to the lower jaw and both jaws are slightly backward relative to the rest of the face. There is a vertical direction of facial growth with a tendency to an increased facial height in the front. This may be tied in with the minimal anterior overbite with a tendency to an edge-to-edge bite. There is minimal protrusion of the upper and lower lips and considerably backward angulation of the upper and lower front teeth. While there is a strong possibility that Alexander will require upper premolar teeth extracted in the future, we have decided to commence orthodontic treatment without extracting any teeth and reassess him once he is approximately six months underway.
>
> Alexander will require expansion of the upper jaw with a quad helix appliance while braces are fitted simultaneously

to commence the alignment of the teeth and begin creation of space for the erupting teeth.

Subsequently, the orthodontist was not satisfied that the desired result was being achieved and referred Alex to an oral and maxilla facial surgeon. Alex had an operation in Canberra to reduce the bone length in his lower jaw and to extend the upper jaw. This brought his upper and lower teeth to a better position above one another for a bite to close appropriately. Despite this effort, his bite would still not close and chewing with molars was impossible. A different surgeon from the same company who had by then moved to Sydney performed another operation using a hip bone graft to build up the right side of his jaw for closure, leaving the left side untouched but with small closure. Alex continued to use his front teeth with an edge-to-edge chew, wearing down these teeth. Ongoing care with his usual dentist included building up the cutting edge of these incisors. Alex was very well behaved for all these arduous procedures.

Alex was to continue with dental problems arising from the facial operations which cut nerves and initiated loosening of his teeth with loss of bone support. In 2015 he received treatment from a prosthodontist involving extraction of loose teeth and trial of bonded acrylic alloy bridges but it did not stop there. The next treatment round occurred while he was incarcerated from 2017 to 2022.

Hope but a set-back

Alex did not understand his intellectual disabilities and kept talking about how he tried at school and undertook studies post-school, as if this would show he does not have intellectual shortcomings. He expressed interest in persisting with literacy and numeracy, for which I entered him in a Canberra Institute of Technology (CIT) program and with private special teachers. Alex made a huge effort in all these activities. Later when he saw his life as heading in the completely wrong direction, he asked me if it was because he did not try hard enough at school. I repeated many times to him that I was proud of him, always getting A+ for effort.

Alex had perspective with his art!

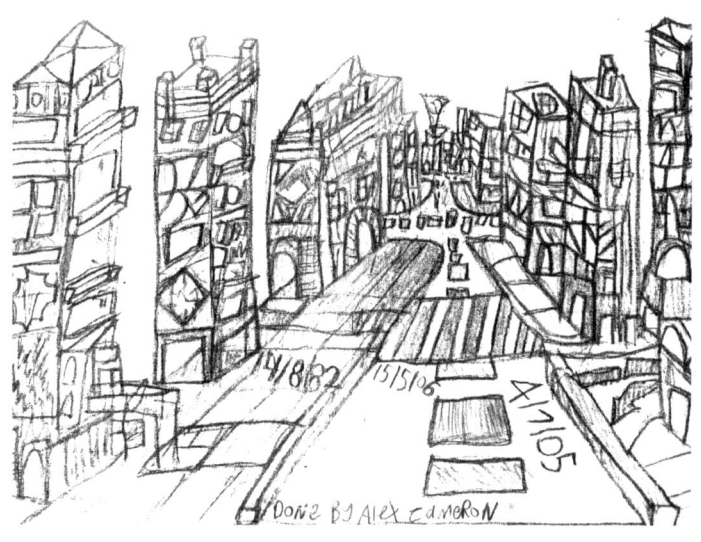

Then something happened in 2007 (Alex aged 25) to destabilise the situation. Alex posed a higher risk of becoming physically violent towards family members. He showed increased manic symptoms especially with excessive shopping during 2007 for clothes and hobbies. He was increasingly unsettled and I scheduled several appointments with his private psychiatrist towards the end of that year. His private psychiatrist made some medicine changes in December 2007. He removed the partial agonist aripiprazole - the medicine he thought was previously beneficial, was added again later and was of contention in the 2017 debacle, but clozapine was retained. I trusted this doctor and optimistically thought things were under control and continued with plans to take our youngest son (then aged 14) on a special holiday as he had tended to miss out on travel once the older boys reached ages at which family holidays were passé. Alex stayed with his father while we were away and the two others were old enough to look after themselves, even if with a bit of mischief. When we returned at the end of January 2008, I realised all was not well with Alex.

Action needed

I tried several more times to get help from the private psychiatrist but by March he said he could not do anymore. I thought Alex was abandoned. The Crisis Team (CATT) began saying it would not do anything because Alex calmed down eventually. The Dual Disability service said Alex did not meet their criteria – oddly something to do with not having a case manager, because this approach said that if you do not have this help, you cannot be eligible for any other help.

I was getting increasingly worried about his outbursts, fearing he could really cause damage and hurt us. The younger boys were on edge. I could call the Crisis Team but if Alex calmed again nothing was done about his potential to keep going into rages. On one occasion the police took him to hospital, the only result of which was an additional prescription of chlorpromazine, an additional antipsychotic.

After three call-outs to the Crisis Team in two weeks of June 2008, there was a horrible evening when he terrorised Donald and bashed both my arms trying to get past me while Donald barricaded himself in his bedroom. That was the worst assault on me at the time and ever. I was black and blue and in pain from the fall I had on the base of my spine while trying to snatch away the cooking pots he was using as weapons. I asked Clive to keep an eye out for the arrival of the police. Ewen, not home that evening, had acted during recent previous crises, holding Alex in a bear hug until he could be safely released. Clive tried to do the same but Alex would not calm down. The event shattered the family for years.

The policeman who arrived decided to charge Alex with assault, explaining he thought it was the only way for me to get help. There ensued a court case requiring a mental health assessment which found him Unfit to Plead. The forensic consultant psychiatrist said that Alex's comments, showing little insight into why he was aggressive, would be in keeping with a diagnosis of some form of organic mental disorder affecting not only cognition but mood and behaviour. The forensic consultant psychiatrist made recommendations about following up the possibility of epilepsy, neuropsychiatric advice and investigation for a chromosome abnormality.

Alex was given bail on condition he not go near me which meant he could not live at home. There was little choice but for Alex to live with his father who had his own health issues.

This lasted a short while with some help on behaviour management from ACT Health but Alex's behaviours were too difficult for his father to manage and he was admitted to the mental health ward. His father obtained a medical certificate for himself recommending he not care for Alex. Charges were eventually dismissed under section 334 of the Crimes Act in August 2008. Nonetheless when Alex could be discharged, we still faced the issue of housing, as I had promised Donald (who was 17 at the time) that he would not have to live under the same roof as Alex again and it was time I tried to move Alex to a place where he could develop independence as an adult.

Aged 26, Alex spent three months in the mental health ward at Canberra Hospital in 2008 from July to October. This was a ward set up prior to the current Adult Mental Health Unit which seems to have a focus on acute cases, seeking to send long-term patients elsewhere. The former adult mental health ward was more accepting of taking Alex's case than the current Adult Mental Health Unit. I went to see him every day. He was a diagnostic dilemma, the hospital psychiatrist Dr A informed me, as if I did not know after all we had been through. Alex could be fractious during his admission but was reasonably well behaved. He could show agitation over small things he did not like. He would frequently hit the sides of his face. He had a tendency to bang my forearm when he was feeling frustrated about something, but not injuring me. His ritualistic and obsessive traits were obvious. He occupied himself with drawing and writing. He was kept in the low dependency area with perhaps one or two uses of seclusion.

He had another bout of pneumonia during this admission. His staying in bed with a giant sweat was not noticed by the nurses and it was on my visit that I was able to bring it to their attention and ask for a doctor. Alex was transferred to a medical ward for IV antibiotic treatment where he recovered. Again, it was suspected to be aspiration pneumonia.

He was prescribed citalopram (serotonin re-uptake inhibitor, antidepressant) during his admission, again considered a possible help for his obsessions and anxiety despite its being ineffective previously. Valproate was added eventually as a mood stabiliser on the advice of the Chief Psychiatrist from the Sydney Children's Hospital on being consulted by Dr A. It was almost immediately effective. The resultant calming made discharge[3] possible – if housing could be organised.

It was thought that there was a synergistic reaction (total more than the sum of individual responses) from valproate and citalopram so there was an argument for retaining the citalopram despite its apparent lack of effect on obsessive symptoms. Further treatment for possible epileptic episodes was discussed but for example, carbamazepine was not a good idea because it would increase the risk of loss of white blood cells on top if this risk from clozapine.

Accommodation change

He was discharged to a respite care share-home for two weeks while we still had no long-term arrangements settled. Thankfully this first move was accomplished with little trouble.

---

[3] He was discharged on clozapine 200mg mornings/300 mg nights, valproate 500 mg bd (100 mg daily) and citalopram 20 mg mornings, coloxyl and senna for constipation induced by clozapine and simvastatin for hypercholesterolaemia. No 5-hydroxtryptophan but I am unclear when this stopped as the supply was a problem.

He was surprisingly adaptable at this stage of his life compared to later times. There was no way public housing would consider providing for him and the case manager unsuccessfully tried several community organisations for a more permanent placement. The situation beyond respite looked hopeless. I then took the risk of purchasing a home for Alex, putting together a deposit and successfully applying for a mortgage. I was lucky to be able to do this. To make it financially viable, however, I had to have two other tenants. The case manager said there would be a long line of people wanting to avail themselves of cheap accommodation. There was no ready access by me to such people even if known to the health unit so I advertised, interviewed and selected otherwise unknown housemates needing cheap accommodation. The ACT Government refused me an exemption from Land Tax, applied to income obtained from property not used as your primary residence, even though I saw myself as supplying what the government should have been providing for Alex.

Alex coped very well after moving from the respite house to his father's, now possible with the successful treatment, and then to the bought townhouse on 1 November 2008. Despite all the changes to his life, he was relatively easy to manage, medicine compliant and cooperative with the people trying to help.

Chapter 3 The good years
2008 - 2017

Despite the disastrous and shocking events, and the hints of enduring undefined problems, medication adjustments at the hospital in 2008 enabled a peaceful discharge and many years of satisfactory community living. The hospital admission enabled a referral to the Dual Disability Unit through which Alex was seen by the expert dual-disability psychiatrist visiting from Sydney from early 2009. He was also referred to a Therapy ACT psychologist and a new consultant psychiatrist, to oversee his care in the community and to liaise with the Sydney visiting doctor. The nature of ongoing contact with either of these professionals was not made explicit to me but I did not chase answers while Alex was doing so well.

The 3-bedroom, two story townhouse that I bought had two courtyards for a pleasant outlook two ways. It had one bathroom but with an extra toilet downstairs, it was suitable for coping with Alex's extended stays in the toilet. It had a big garage with a bench for his art and crafts.

Enjoying life

Alex was able to gradually resume many interests. He resumed his work at the Koomarri Association which ran businesses using supervised workshops for those with disabilities. He played tennis in the Special Olympics, participated in a drama group, went bike riding and played ten pin bowling. He worked at Pack 'N' Post at Koomarri Association three days per week, where he had a reputation for hard work (once you could get him away from distracting habits and rituals). He was tried at a variety of tasks, including rag sorting, soldering, packaging of airline headsets and collation of documents into folders. He continued his art and craft on other days.

Japan

The first plane we had to take was from Canberra to Sydney then from Sydney to the Toyama Airport in Japan. At the Airport we also had our own Drama shirts on to wear on the trip.

In Japan on the bus we had traveled a really much long way from the Airport to where we had to stay while in Japan. On the bus we also had some Japanese food to eat. It was some rice with some little tasty dumplings and nice little bits of pâtés and pasties While in Japan I had been in my group rehearsing my Skeleton play in the Dark. We had done our play twice, once in a school and once in the building that we did our play in. In one of the days in Japan we had a walk through some parks that had some very interesting things like little cemented monument statues. Even a big long high up Japanese character Monument. Some of the places we went through were really good, some we even ate Japanese ice-cream somewhere to eat while out of the hot sun.

The drama group, comprising past students of Black Mountain school and managed by a generous volunteer, took him on travels: one trip to Japan and another to India. His life seemed relatively happy and productive.

Alex loved to write either by hand or typing into his computer. Particularly when he felt it was hard to get people to listen to him verbally, he turned to written communication. An example is his report on his drama trip to Japan, an excerpt of which is in the box. I include this piece written while in non-manic mood for comparison with later writings.

He was proud enough of his new home to invite old school friends to visit. He remained very loyal to his school friends even when he had not been able to see them for years. One school friend in particular took Alex out several times, kept in touch with me if not Alex over the years and came to his memorial service in 2023.

There was none of the violent outbursts from before the hospital admission. There were setbacks in the form of increased agitation and distress over minor matters such as ants in the kitchen, but there was more help on hand. The case manager schooled Alex on ringing for help himself if he thought he was out of control but I do not know how well this worked. He might have commenced an out of control event slowly enough to recognise what was happening at this stage of his life.

Alex had more visits from the community health team and sometimes was treated with PRN – such as diazepam or olanzapine to calm him. A cleaning service was arranged. The case manager arranged meals through Meals on Wheels which would not deliver because of perceived risks, but a pick-up was arranged. I read about this help in Alex's Progress Notes years later. I would have liked to have been kept better informed at the time.

Medication monitoring

In the summer of 2008-09 Alex was not managing the heat well which could have been associated with his clozapine. He seemed over-sedated most of the time. The community psychiatrist was keen to reduce the dose of clozapine to the lowest effective dose to also minimise side effects such as an increased appetite for carbohydrates. He gradually reduced the clozapine until Alex developed more fractiousness which occurred below 225 mg per day. I read incidentally later that his case manager interpreted his inability to sleep, with his claim he saw something in his cupboard at night, as hallucinating when on a low dose at this time. Again, here was information not shared with me at the time, when it would have been appropriate with a guardian.

Aripiprazole 10 mg was added again in his regimen in February 2009 which might have been more necessary given Alex's lower dosage of clozapine. Valproate was increased to 1500 mg daily. Citalopram was dropped by this stage but I am not sure when.

Interest in a broader diagnosis

Alex first saw the Sydney dual disability psychiatrist in late February 2009. In his report to the community psychiatrist, this doctor commented on the different tests of cognitive functioning undertaken in 1989 (7 years) - upper end of low average, to 1994 (11 years) - low average, to 1998 (16 years) – mental retardation. I had never been clear about how to interpret these results as Alex's anxieties increased as he aged too, interfering with his comfort with being tested. Also, his extent and kind of medication at each testing was not recorded and I thought perhaps that he was not medicated at all at the time of the 1998 test. The Sydney dual disability psychiatrist described the results as a "catastrophic decline" in cognition.

The dual disability psychiatrist asked for genetic testing. This was done by ACT Genetics but this laboratory interpreted the doctor's interest as an effort to relate genetics with depression. Depression was not actually one of Alex's symptoms of note and he displayed amazing energy and effort to keep going despite what he was put through. The real question was about relating Alex's neurological issues such as his intellectual disabilities with a genetic cause. I think the misdirection came from a mention of familial depression as if the only interest was in inherited genes. Unsurprisingly, the chromosomal analysis did not identify anything. The exome analysis which was eventually done years later was not an available technique in 2009.

Alex's diagnoses from early childhood had been difficult, and variable, depending on the views of the particular professionals whose advice we sought. As indicated, he was being regarded as a diagnostic dilemma exhibiting overlapping syndromes of Tourette Syndrome, Attention Deficit Disorder, Obsessive Compulsive Disorder and poor impulse control in conjunction with intellectual disability and afferent schizoid symptoms, and possibly epilepsy. His intellectual disability was diagnosed and discussed as possibly deteriorating with age. As a child, autism was specifically eliminated based on the dominant diagnostic features of the 1980s (earlier visiting psychiatrist from Sydney) and thus interventions for autism were never made. Manic symptoms were not medically identified in childhood.

Limits on retrospective analysis

One cannot get a reliable list of medications and timing of changes from Alex's Patient Progress reports. I went back to these reports because type and dosage of medication became increasingly important from 2017 onwards. It was also important to have a record of responsiveness and residual behavioural problems associated with his regimen at a particular time. I noted that from 2008 to 2017 Alex was adequately managed on clozapine 225 mg daily (a low dose), aripiprazole (increased to 15 mg daily) and valproate 1500 mg daily. Sertraline seems to have restarted in April 2014, increased to 100 mg in August 2014 and noted as still 100 mg daily May 2015 but possibly increased to 150 mg daily in 2016. Its purpose was to address obsessive compulsive disorder (OCD) but had no effect on Alex's behaviours labelled OCD. These reports were from within the health system including from the community clozapine clinic.

The reports originating in the clozapine clinic list some of his medication, but not all, when I know that he was taking other medication. There were omissions in his taking of sertraline and aripiprazole and various dosages of sertraline were given. It might be important to have an accurate record for this antidepressant for the purpose of including adverse effects from sertraline among the theories for Alex's destabilisation in 2017. I reiterate, when Alex was a child, sertraline seemed to be the cause of more extreme erratic behaviour in Alex.

Perhaps for the purposes of the clozapine clinic they were not interested in all his medicines. Clozapine was listed accurately all the time it appears. As well as hit and miss with other psychiatric medication, any medications prescribed by his GP were not listed in these reports. Thus, there is no record with a full and accurate list of Alex's medications over time. I provide details of Alex's medication with dosages throughout this story where I have the information because it is integral to explaining the medical carelessness and mistakes.

Doctors used the wording that he was *historically* violent. This implies this behaviour was unrelenting and not related to variability or adequacy of medication. They seemed not to be able to discriminate about dates and circumstances for nuanced communication to any subsequent professional readers of his records. It was possible that they had limited access to records, perhaps seeing only the Crisis Team reports, not the monthly clozapine clinic reports. Alex had some difficulties, but his stable profile at this time should have been recorded as his best self to which treatments after setbacks should have been aimed.

Challenges

Swelling in Alex's lower legs and ankles was very noticeable for a few years at this stage. This was in combination with the petechiae (brown-purple spots) on his lower legs which seemed to be due to minor bleeding in the dermis. I had asked the private psychiatrist earlier if they were due to clozapine but he was doubtful. He did not suggest any treatment and seemed unconcerned. The case manager arranged an emergency GP appointment for Alex in 2009. The GP was not concerned and a little later a health worker thought the swelling was resolving. Any connection between the spots (leakiness of capillaries perhaps) and oedema was not mentioned.

The excellent case manager who oversaw his discharge in 2008 and transition to community was moved elsewhere, which upset Alex as he grew to be fond of her. She had maintained contact and saw him at his monthly clozapine clinic attendances. He had several supportive nurses and supports during his stay at the townhouse. On special occasions family friends would visit.

I visited him at least three times per week, attended to the garden and any cleaning not getting done. I tried to make sure he was getting good meals. On his workdays I telephoned using the landline early in the morning to make sure he was awake. This annoyed one of his first housemates who liked to sleep in! Alex managed the bus from his new suburb to get to work on his own.

I had variable success with the housemates and their ability to live with Alex and not create new challenges. I had to recruit new ones a few times. I was finding it very tiring looking after two homes but kept it going until 2010. Then, with a suspicion that one flatmate had friends bringing drugs I became uneasy. A newly separated father as a tenant wanting to have his children at the house on weekends was a further complication. The father then complained about a housemate loudly boasting of his sexual exploits. It was not looking like a good environment for Alex either.

Another living arrangement

Ewen, then Donald, moved out of our home by 2010, while Clive continued to live with me. I reconsidered Alex's living arrangements and my abilities. I thought that he might be better living closer to me but still be independent. I wanted him to have opportunities for gradually learning more skills for coping on his own. A suitable arrangement might be possible with Donald away from home now. A house with a granny flat would be ideal. After rejecting the idea of building onto our current home, I decided to rent out the townhouse I bought earlier for Alex, sell our home of 21 years and purchase a new place with capacity to allow Alex his own space close to me. I knew making such a big change for Alex was risky.

However, despite an initial upset when told of the move, Alex coped with moving back to his father's while I waited for settlement on the new house and renovated a lower level for his new flat. He came to really love his flat and when he was held in mental health facilities later, he kept extolling its virtues and regretting not being there. Even when living away from him, Alex would love to spend weekends with his father who regarded him as good company at this time. Alex accompanied his father on hobby outings such as for model trains and enjoyed helping him by making tea and sandwiches.

There were no issues warranting crisis help during 2011-2013. Alex made complaints of frequently feeling the need to urinate, not necessarily frequent urination, and I kept an eye on his swollen legs. He began putting on weight but not excessively so. In December 2014, he was admitted to Hospital in the Home for treatment of cellulitis in the right lower leg. He was also diagnosed with fungal infection between the toes. Of interest for being able to consider and discuss his medicine regime coincident with moods and behaviours later, the hospital recorded at this time daily clozapine 225 mg, aripiprazole 15 mg, sertraline 100mg and valproate 1500 mg. Of significance for what happened in 2017 is the record of Alex being on aripiprazole. This hospital record should have been accessible by all doctors from within the system!

Alex could be frustrated in this period but mostly without losing control. He exhibited agitation when trying to get ready for a particular deadline but peak agitation level was not over the top and calming down was relatively easy. He would seek time in his bedroom to calm down by himself. The worst event over this nine-year period to 2017 was property damage with a one-off hole punched in his bedroom door. Alex became extra frustrated while a carer was waiting for him or felt he was not going to get his lift to tennis perhaps.

Getting on with daily living

During his time in his independent flat his usual activities centred on domestic duties, attending to his tasks such as shopping and medical appointments and pursuing his multiple hobbies, including prolific art works. By 2016, Alex was learning to cut short some activities if running out of time to get somewhere. Inability to factor in extra time he needed to do various tasks and persistence with his self-listed activities to be done, regardless of the clock, meant he often had to forego outings or his work and often led to frustrations. Some workers could be flexible but many times they had to leave Alex before any outing or activity. Alex's evenings became so taken up with meals, medications, toileting and teeth cleaning that he was getting to bed later and later in 2016-17, but without going to work he had more opportunities to sleep in.

His ability to discuss doing things another way was impaired by obsessions and his need to employ his own control over operations. It was getting increasingly difficult to teach him new approaches as he sought self-agency, but he was not getting physically violent in his objections. Alex still went to the toilet a lot and spent an excessive time there.

He would wash dishes, clean his teeth or undertake other exercises with more vigour and repetitive action than was required. He would not seem to know when to stop and not learn from worn out toothbrushes or broken vacuum cleaner heads etc. From about 2015 Alex wanted to spend more time in mainstream company so that he thought more about mainstream work and giving up his sporting activities which were with disability groups. He wanted to stack shelves in the supermarket for example.

Alex began avoiding work in 2015. He looked forward to his outings with support workers to pursue his walking and photography but not to doing things with others with disabilities. In 2016 he had great outings with his Health Unit Recovery Officer. Alex still had difficulties getting ready on time, and often wore inappropriate clothing for hot days. Overall, these were some of the happiest days in his life.

Alex kept a calendar on which to write his appointments and planned trips. He would often remind me of his appointments.

He could manage buses himself but needed help when a new route was required. He was sometimes worried about other passengers and the looks he found suspicious. He began walking to and from the bus interchange to avoid at least one leg of his bus journey to work. His love of art and craft, taking photographs, making files on his computer and ten-pin bowling continued.

He walked with a hunched-forward gait, walking rapidly and in curved paths. He could charge ahead of everyone, carry home big bags of shopping and seemed strong and robust.

He spent a lot of time thinking and shopping for family birthdays and Christmas presents. He liked to make his own cards for presents and was creative with use of foam sheeting to make boxes and models of buildings etc. He made a modular road system for his remote control car using painted foam board sheets.

Alex would rarely sit through an entire movie or music recording in one sitting and would not play anything loudly or for long. He could shop for more things than he needed, liking collections: clothes which perhaps were not ever worn, video tapes not watched, books not read, huge number of CDs for photograph storage, batteries that would be depleted in storage before required. After my remonstrance on his massive shopping binge in 2007 (mania), Alex took to checking with me about large purchases. There was more control.

He would attend to showering and shaving with verbal prompts from me. He also needed prompts to stop showering and stop drying. He attended to his own clothes washing but was less interested in washing sheets and towels. He was resistant to housecleaning, saying it would just get dirty again. He had pre-NDIS fortnightly floor cleaning from a community organisation but he told them not to come again when there was a period of new people coming each time.

Donald had to move home again for a short while and this presented no problems given the time since the 2007 incident and Alex's stability and ease with which we all got on with him in these years. Alex saw Donald and Clive for evening meals until he chose to take his plate back to his flat to eat there.

Alex was always keen to be helpful with property and garden chores. He regarded putting the bins out at the gutter as his job for example. He often visited his father to help him out at his home. Alex continued to join his father for outings related to his father's hobbies of model trains, gemstones, photography and fishing. He was well behaved on these outings and sought to be helpful, for example setting up tables for the model railways show.

Alex was compliant with his clozapine routine, often taking himself to the pathology agent monthly for blood sampling. He would often ring his recovery officer himself to ask about being taken to his next clozapine appointment. He took charge of his own Webster[4] packs and did not need supervision to ensure his tablets were taken.

He behaved well in shops. He did his own supermarket shopping for breakfast and lunch for several years and by 2017

---

[4] Pharmacy certified blister pack comprising compartments with the prescribed medicines sorted according to time and date for administration.

wanted to do his own evening meals, but this did not prove a good step. His evening meals under his control became layered creations using frozen meals sandwiched with lashings of mustard, tomato sauce and BBQ sauce, adding perhaps tartare sauce for good measure. He did not have a weight problem while he had several sport activities, walked a lot and had my evening meals without the add-ons that he was introducing in 2017.

The introduction of the NDIS

A National Disability Insurance Scheme (NDIS) program[5] for Alex commenced in early 2017 which was very much welcomed by me. Alex loved the chances of companionship it provided but not disability labels. An NDIS Plan setting out what funds could pay for and how much was approved and a program of support workers commenced. I selected an experienced organisation for a support coordinator and fund manager. Alex enjoyed getting to know his support coordinator on several outings and they had excellent rapport. I had many discussions about developing his supports program and highlighted learning to cook and joining in community activities. Sustained relationships were made between Alex and these workers.

A learning problem became evident once we tried skill building with the cooking support. Attempts to use NDIS

---

[5] The promising new Australian NDIS commenced early in the ACT with a trial in 2014. When the scheme was available more broadly Alex was able to apply successfully to be a participant in 2016 with implementation in 2017. National implementation was not achieved until 2020.

funded disability support to improve this meal preparation failed when he ignored their help. Alex only wanted people to watch him do what he thought should be done and was not open to any alternatives suggested. Support Workers ended up staying in the background while Alex did what he wanted. The support coordinator found a psychologist who might be able to analyse what Alex was thinking and doing when offered opportunities to learn new skills. We were optimistically working on issues.

I thought we had arrived at optimal treatment for Alex and he would be set up for a good life. I began to think about what might be his next step to be even more independent and to be able to cope as I aged.

2017 was the year plans were shattered.

Chapter 4 Misjudgement and overreaction
September 2017 – January 2018

2017 commenced for us with an atmosphere of uncertainty and imminent change. My closest sister in Melbourne was severely ill and by April was diagnosed with ovarian cancer, the cancer that is not detected until it is possibly too late. I was heading for retirement after twenty-eight years in the public service in the Commonwealth Department of Health. Alex had been turning away from his usual interests and his position with Koomarri Pack 'N' Post, declaring he did not want to identify with only disability groups, not that he called them that. The introduction of the National Disability Insurance Scheme (NDIS), and consequently the introduction of support workers, had caused him to uncover the use of the word disability in association with himself for the first time. We had not discussed why he had been only doing work and sports with disability groups until then. Alex just accepted that was what he did but did not see himself as having disabilities. Thus, there were signs of change from Alex.

My changes might have worried him, for example, about my retirement. He articulated fears it meant I was becoming too old to look after myself and he would have to look after me.

He was very protective and wanted to exercise agency in household matters. He wanted to see himself as the man of the house, to take control. He was always desperate to show his abilities. He did not want me to die. He did not think about himself dying at this stage.

I realised early in 2017 that Alex needed attention to his physical health issues. Of concern were:

- symptoms of epileptic *absences* (petit-mal) – a new form commencing in 2015 and increasing in frequency
- intermittent and unexplained vomiting – not all events witnessed by me
- venous incompetence in both legs – swelling in his legs progressively increasing, exacerbated by contracting cellulitis two years previously.

Alex's GP had dismissed my worries about Alex's legs earlier. I took Alex to a new GP who explored carefully each issue on my list. Alex saw a Canberra neurologist, for the *absences* and a vascular surgeon for his leg veins. The surgeon said there was insufficient reason to intervene with vein surgery and Alex should wear compression stockings and raise his legs when possible.

The neurologist increased the dose of valproate, the anticonvulsant that Alex had been taking since 2008 as a mood stabiliser to 2000 mg. My records are that the increase in valproate came in September 2017.

The GP explored the potential for acid reflux and ulcers as part of the vomiting story. No ulcer was found but proton inhibitors were prescribed for reducing stomach acid. But why these small vomits? I had observed Alex overeat at a meal and then partially vomit so I assumed this fullness was the cause. I tried to guide Alex into better meal sizes. I encouraged him to take his regular tablets at least a half hour after meals to reduce the chance of him regurgitating them, on the assumption that his stomach would be more settled.

Another destabilisation

It was coincident with the increase in valproate and vomiting from September to October that we noticed changes in behaviour in Alex, although there had been a minor incident in 2016, which had quickly resolved. He showed aggression in late 2017 which was most unusual compared to his behaviour since 2008, aggression which increased in frequency and increased in severity in these weeks. He wanted to control the way I was answering a sales nuisance phone call one night, grabbing the receiver from me and kicking me. Then one evening I went downstairs to his separate kitchenette to see if I could help his attempt to cook. He threw the burnt contents of a frypan with hot oil at me. Luckily the oil was not still at cooking temperature and it hit my sleeve, not my bare skin. I was sufficiently worried nonetheless to want to seek help from the health sector. Alex was showing reduced control and I wanted to prevent another episode such as in 2008.

I can see my mistakes in retrospect. If only I had not taken action in expecting help from the health system, the ghastly progression of events, the inexorable journey to his early death, would not have occurred. I certainly needed help. Primarily I needed help to make sure that Alex was eating properly, that his vomiting was more closely monitored and that he got a reasonable amount of sleep. If the NDIS had the capacity to provide emergency support, it would have been preferable to get such help in-home rather than via the hospital admission. Through asking for help from the health services I unwittingly set in motion the worst years imaginable for Alex.

In Early October I sought help from the local Mental Health Unit where Alex had attended each month as part of his clozapine supervision. My request was not regarded as urgent and the psychiatrist, Dr A, who normally saw Alex in the clozapine clinic, was on leave. I spoke to Alex's disability support coordinator who investigated alternative accommodation potential given increased risk to family.

In reflecting on what had changed for Alex to bring this about, I considered further whether the vomiting gave rise to incomplete ingestion of his medicine. I thought this unlikely from my questioning of Alex on the timing of vomits and small volumes of each vomit, but I could not rule it out.

I tried to explore whether the increase in valproate dose for his petit mal seizures had a negative effect. I checked both the US Federal Drug Administration and Australia's Adverse Drug Reactions Committee websites and found reports of increased aggression for the combination of valproate with clozapine. This was at a low frequency but it was still possible and had an increased likelihood in males. I did not consider at this time whether sertraline was the culprit as Alex had been prescribed this for a while prior to the destabilisation in 2017. Dr A had been increasing the dosage from 2016 to 2017. It was difficult to make a temporal association between a high dose of sertraline and the increased aggression.

When I was eventually able to talk to Dr A, he was interested and when he had a chance, he reduced Alex's valproate dose but the idea was never fully explored in the hospitals. I kept bringing this up throughout the next five years. At times my bringing this idea to other doctors' attention was met with curt dismissal. "Don't be silly, valproate reduces aggression, it does not cause it" they said. Undeterred, I uncovered a mechanism for it to be a reasonable explanation. Valproate increases the metabolism of clozapine resulting in decreases in available clozapine and thus decreases the effectiveness for a given dose of clozapine. Alex was on a low dose of clozapine meaning anything affecting blood levels could more easily affect him clinically. If a clinician does not connect lowering of blood levels of an antipsychotic to increased aggression, then of course the clinician does not consider the significance of this.

The first blocks to appropriate treatment

I was not able to see Dr A until 3 November having begged for an earlier appointment to no avail. Then, Dr A was so surprised at the different Alex he saw, that he wanted to arrange for a hospital admission the same day. Alex did not want to go! Workers from Mental Health visited home and talked him into packing a bag. About three hours later he was admitted to hospital. His health and life course were never going to recover.

I went into the assessment area in which they held him at the hospital. The doctor on duty chatted and went through his medication list orally. I alerted them to the omission of aripiprazole (the partial agonist antipsychotic) which Alex has been taking for several years in conjunction with clozapine. The doctor said he did not have that on his list but I was very firm. He did not say he did not believe me and neither did he say he would check. The next day I took in Alex's Webster medication pack to prove that I was right but there was a different doctor on duty. This second doctor pleasantly took the packs but gave no commitments.

When I finally obtained copies of the notes these doctors made, I could read no reference at all to my saying Alex was also on aripiprazole, even though my visit itself was documented. The same hospital had on record the use of aripiprazole when he was treated for his cellulitis in 2014. In this instance in 2017, had they no access to mental health records, or perhaps they relied on only the clozapine clinic notes but those were never rigorously prepared regarding medication. Whatever was behind the initial mistake, another chance to rectify the omission was lost. In his Health Progress Notes there is a hospital pharmacist's note made a few days into Alex's 2017 admission requesting a medicine review because Alex's Webster packs did not match his charted medication, but there is no record of action taken.

Even if the health record system were at the root cause, the fundamental mistake was not listening to me. I told them they had the error in his medicine list. And I had been naive enough to think they would rectify the situation during his stay.

I only found out that the hospital had completely failed to prescribe aripiprazole when the community pharmacist, who had habitually included aripiprazole in the packs, rang me to ask why it was omitted post discharge two weeks later. The hospital was too casual over administering correct medication, had unreliable records and displayed poor practice in its failure to listen to me, his prime carer. The hospital psychiatrist caring for Alex in the ward, Dr B, had not checked. Dr B was responsible for starting Alex on the whole horror story.

In a response to my complaint to the Health Commission I made in March 2018, the hospital administration denied that Dr B had made any mistake. Misrepresentations and defensiveness occurred within the system about failures in communication systems and shortcomings professionally of doctors. Dr C made a note in the Progress Notes later that the omission of aripiprazole was an accident. Is it any wonder I kept questioning and trying to understand the medical justifications for Alex's treatments?

A failing system

There was no way back on a better track but I did not know that at the time. I kept thinking we could overcome the obstacles. I will labour over some details in the next stages of the story because descriptions of this descent into hell is important. It will help to explain why Alex was heading for a disastrous situation.

Three days after being taken to Royal Canberra Hospital (6 November) Alex was held in the High Dependency Unit, which is standard practice when the patient is in an assessment phase. Dr B told me they did not like the pressure to take him. It seemed to me they did not really assess him. I was told that they thought he did not have any mental illness but just suffered from behaviour problems due to intellectual disability. Further, I was told that the Adult Mental Health Unit is an acute ward with no capacity to take time over what was wrong with Alex. Under sufferance they would ask the Tribunal for a two weeks' Psychiatric Treatment Order (PTO) in order to admit him as an involuntary patient. After that he had to go. The Mental Health Tribunal of the ACT Civil and Administrative Tribunal made a PTO which gave the Chief Psychiatrist power to detain Alex for care despite his desire to go home.

Alex was in shock at the treatment in such an austere and strict place and was not likely to improve in that environment, especially with one of his significant medicines withdrawn. The High Dependency Unit is kept as a low stimulus environment but sometimes playing in the courtyard with a ball was arranged or films would be shown. Patients had their own rooms with bathrooms with contact with other patients made in the dining and lounge area. Alex had no idea what mental illness was and found the other patients frightening. He saw as a threat those who were psychotic and mumbling. Unless a nurse came into their area, patient initiated contact was made by knocking on a heavy security door and waiting. Only through this process could a hot drink be received for example. Alex yelled at me to get him out. But the situation got worse.

On 14 November, I was hurriedly shown two community group houses as potential accommodation for Alex at the end of the two weeks. One contained a group about to move to another house. I knew this was bad for Alex who did not like change. The other house was unclean but had reasonable space and friendly residents. The care workers were unknown to Alex and I knew nothing about the organisations responsible for each house. I was to discover that neither organisation understood Alex's dual disability and that one of the organisations was owned/managed by the husband of the "Case Worker" who selected these houses for showing. I had no time. Faced with homelessness or having him back home with me, I chose from the two houses shown to me, the community home whose occupants would at least not be about to transfer. This Case Worker appointed by the Mental Health Unit on the day he was admitted to the hospital knew nothing about Alex and nothing about his intellectual disabilities even if they knew something about mental illness.

On the two-week mark, 17 November, Alex was expected to cope in the community. There was no discharge plan. Alex was not given any preparation for this discharge to a community house. He could not understand why he could not go home with me. The Case Worker insisted on picking him up from the hospital while I collected some of Alex's furniture from home, so I have no idea what they said to him in the process. He put on a loud aggressive tantrum on being dropped off. I could see he was unwell and asked for him to be taken back to hospital. They refused. Not knowing Alex, they might have assumed that his behaviour was normal. We managed to get him inside and calmer.

18 November: Alex calmed down and seemed to be pleased to be introduced to the residents. I took him home to allow him to select some items to take back to the house. He returned to the house uneventfully. I was more positive.

Involvement of police

19 November: I made the mistake of thinking I should stay away from the house to let Alex settle in with his new companions and carers. No one had explained they relied on residents having mobile phones. The landline was not working. Alex did not have a mobile phone and did not know how to use one. He tried to ring me by borrowing one from a carer but he got frustrated and struck out at the carer who protected himself with his arm. A resident got scared and rang the police. By the time the police arrived Alex was in the kitchen where there was a knife nearby on the bench. Of course, the police went for the knife, but Alex objected to someone taking property that was not theirs. In the ensuing scuffle, Alex's hand was cut and they held him on the ground, handcuffed him and took him to the police station remand Watch House. Alex was not receptive to cooperation with police while he was ill with inadequate medication!

Neither the police nor the carers rang me, his guardian, until the next day when the house staff rang me. Alex had missed his medication that night. He had tried to take his medication before he left the house but the police would not let him. Why the carer had not thought to ring me himself before the furore, once Alex had expressed the desire to contact me, I have no idea. I could have been there in ten minutes. I could only imagine how terrified Alex was.

20 November: Alex appeared before Magistrate Theakson. I was daunted and anxious in that environment so I expect Alex went through something worse. He was charged with assault and resisting arrest. The appointed duty solicitor for Alex told

the magistrate incorrectly that Alex lived in an aged care home. It seemed he had no real interest in Alex's real circumstances. Alex was given bail on condition he did not harm the named person again. The health liaison officer was very pleased with herself in being able to tell me Alex was not psychotic (which he wasn't on the basis he had no paranoia and hallucinations). She thought she was giving me good news but I knew it meant that Alex would get no help. I spoke to the duty solicitor outside court to explain the risk, but given no evidence of psychosis according to professional assessment, nothing was done about his need for treatment and I was forced to take Alex home again.

I engaged a lawyer for Alex so he would be properly represented.

Incompetence revealed

24 November: I had an appointment with Dr A, who defended the need for the hospital admission. He admitted the hospital discharge was bad practice and that psychiatry should be interested in problems outside psychoses. On the other hand, he was also of the mindset that Alex symptoms outside paranoia and hallucinations were due to "behaviour" from learned bad responses. He had not aired this opinion in all the time he was Alex's clozapine clinic doctor. He expressed disapproval that aripiprazole was removed from Alex's medicines as if it were a therapeutic decision. He nonetheless recommended that an alternative (quetiapine) antipsychotic/mood stabiliser could be trialled and noted he disagreed with the increased dose by the hospital of

antidepressant sertraline because it could increase anxiety. However, he did not change it.

Surprisingly he chose this moment to express concern about Alex being historically treated with clozapine as he said, "It is a very strong antipsychotic". He had overseen Alex's treatment with this for years and had not raised the issue previously. He had known Alex since he was admitted in early 2008 to the then Mental Health Unit at the hospital.

At a later interview Dr A completely contradicted himself regarding the omission of aripiprazole when Alex had been admitted to hospital at the beginning of November. He changed the story to acknowledging accidental omission.

Dr A introduced quetiapine, the different antipsychotic/mood stabiliser and reduced, in two stages, the dosage of valproate (anticonvulsant, mood stabiliser). It was not immediately obvious that these changes were helpful. Quetiapine had only been successful in making Alex oversleep, with greater irritability in wake periods. There was no plan for Alex to be seen by Dr A in the near future. Alex had to wait until January for an appointment with the neurologist, to consider a different anticonvulsant. The earliest he could see the Sydney dual-disability psychiatrist with intellectual disability expertise again in Canberra was January 2018 too.

From late November to early December, Alex stayed at home with his behaviour variable, but at times explosive. I limited my contact with him in case I accidentally triggered him. The Mental Health Unit provided what they thought was support, in the form of several brief visits by the new case manager and/or other staff. The case manager aggravated Alex with questions about his behaviour, questioning him as if he had insight. She continued to misunderstand intellectual disability and his lack of self-awareness of mental illness, suggesting he do mindfulness exercises! I had to abruptly leave the room when she said this because I was going to be very rude.

I could not cope

One day when Alex went into a rage during the case manager's visit, the team called an ambulance but the ambulance officer refused to take Alex as he was calmer by the time it arrived. He has to be seen to be a risk to himself or others for action to be taken under the Mental Health Act.

11 December: This was another day I regretted. I called the police this time when Alex refused to stop pushing the mental health team members and thumping their car. For work reasons, the team members did not want to talk to the police about any assault. Using Alex's threat on me of the previous night 10 December, waving a heavy metal grating off the top of my stove, police charged Alex with an assault in addition to the November charge. My youngest son, Clive was able to physically restrain Alex while he calmed down that night. Alex had not struck anyone. No one was hurt.

Just as I had a good experience with police in 2008 when they helped me get medical help for Alex, I thought it would be constructive this time. At that time, the police said they would charge him so that I would get help after the health sector abandoned me. All I achieved this time was a continuation of the poor treatment of Alex.

Could the court help?

12 December: There is a mix up about the time Alex was due to appear before the magistrate. Clive my youngest son came with me. We waited all morning and were told we had time to take a lunch break. When we returned Alex had already been brought in and was dealt with. We waited until the end of the session that day to be able to ask the Associate what happened and to explain that we thought that the relevant information was not being brought before the Magistrate. We found out that Alex reacted with rage in front of the Magistrate and was placed in the Alexander Maconochie Centre (ACT Gaol) to reappear at a later date. His Honour assessed that as Alex was not in a state representing an *acute* risk, he could not commit him to a mental institution.

The Associate advised each of us to write letters to the Magistrate. Clive was placed in the witness box when Alex's case next appeared before the Magistrate to give evidence that we were faced with a new acute situation with Alex. The essential point to be made was that Alex had definitely not presented consistently over the years with the same behaviours as now. We had had peace since 2008 and there had been good times before that 2007-2008 disruption. Alex was presenting with a destabilisation, warranting medical care, not dismissal based on the assumption he is simply always like this. His Honour directed Alex to hospital under section 309 of the Crimes Act 1900 (ACT) (assessment of mental health).

It was only Clive's evidence that was able to persuade his Honour to transport Alex to a mental health facility. The professional advice to the court was that Alex was not suffering from an acute condition. The alternative to going back to hospital was the ACT Gaol Alexander Maconochie Centre. Theoretically we had the better option at the hospital with health care, but he was under Dr B.

Bad to worse

13 – 21 December: Dr B persisted under a bias that Alex was not mentally ill but had "behaviours", the consequences of which made Alex even sicker. Dr B told me they consulted with Dr A, who perhaps they assumed, really knew Alex. They said they had strong doubts that the diagnosis of schizophrenia was right and wanted to take him off clozapine. We had a hospital doctor biased against Alex having any mental illness in collusion with a community doctor with sudden doubts about Alex's diagnosis and treatment. They were puzzled and worried about Alex exhibiting odd behaviour whilst being on a "strong" antipsychotic, clozapine. This hardly promised to be a well thought-through medical decision to remove clozapine, as if the previous years since he was fifteen or sixteen on clozapine was under incompetent psychiatrists (Sydney and Canberra) who did not know what they were doing.

Dr A reportedly said he had never seen symptoms of schizophrenia so perhaps Alex didn't need clozapine. This is a common mistake in patients who see no symptoms while taking a medication so they stop taking it against medical advice and do not see themselves becoming sick again. I had never previously known a doctor to produce this kind of logic.

When Dr B told me of this decision to take Alex off clozapine, I thought that Alex was at least in the right place for observation. The Adult Mental Health Unit showed no such capacity. It seemed that the doctors were not paying attention to changing symptoms. Nurses' notes reported no hallucination, paranoia nor delusions, which was probably accurate at the early stages. but neither did they recognise Alex's emerging symptoms suggestive of mania such as his increased talking and the socialisation which was actually out of the ordinary. Alex now had no antipsychotics, noting he had the aripiprazole omitted earlier. Withdrawing clozapine should be associated with close observation during a slow reduction of dosing[6]. I do not know whether Alex's withdrawal was too rapid giving rise to his rebound. I observed that the Adult Mental Health Unit was not closely monitoring what staff did not recognise as psychotic symptoms.

Alex was kept there involuntarily with a combination of the judicial and mental health processes. The Tribunal made another PTO from 15 December to 27 December when an extension was made until March. On 21 December the Magistrate made a Restriction Order taking away the orders under section 309 of the Crimes Act. Pursuant to this, Alex was given bail requiring he comply with his PTO and he remain at the AMHU. This felt like a relief but Alex was not clear of the judicial process yet and there was no promise of help from the hospital.

---

[6] If abrupt discontinuation of clozapine is necessary the patient should be observed carefully for return of psychotic symptoms, which may recur quickly, and withdrawal symptoms related to cholinergic rebound such as vomiting and agitation.
https://www.hcpinfo.clozaril.co.uk/-/media/clozarilcouk/pdf/factsheet-discontinuing-treatment.pdf

5 January 2018: At a family meeting, labelled a discharge meeting because the hospital was really planning a discharge before the end of the month, there was no mention of Alex possibly relapsing, no recognition of manic symptoms, and it seemed they were only looking for hallucinations and delusions. Alex was moved to the Low Dependency Unit under Dr B's judgement that he was doing far better by then with clozapine blood levels reduced to zero. They were pleased with his elevated mood in conjunction with more socialisation and articulation of creative ideas. I was sceptical, but of course if he briefly had reduced aggression that could only be good, right? I reported my concerns that he was not back to normal on 9 January. They did not know what he was like when well. I did.

12 January: I attended the Friday hospital meeting to discuss discharge, what the NDIS support required and what might be sought from the Sydney expert when he visited 19 January. Dr B reported on this day that Alex had no psychotic symptoms at all! Dr B asserted that Alex was ready to go home but they were interested in what the Sydney expert might have to say, which was an attitude we were grateful for.

The hospital had made him sicker

I went to see Alex after the meeting and found his elevated mood which included play acting with jumping on his bed as an imaginary character rather disturbing. Was he delusional now as well? I was told by staff that Alex had required a sedative that morning to try to keep him calm. Surely that does not match with someone supposedly ready for discharge. I made further observations over the weekend and, not believing I would get any relevant immediate attention, I waited until Monday morning to contact Dr B. I emailed Dr B about my concerns from weekend observations showing more extreme behaviours. I used email for communication a lot because calls were often not successful, perhaps because staff were too busy.

Before that email could have been read on Monday 15 January, Dr B rang me to report that Alex had been throwing things and had used a chair to break a reinforced window. He had been moved back to HDU! Nurse/doctor observations, in focussing on hallucinations and thought disorder, completely ignored his heightened energy. It can take a while for a full emergence of disease symptoms after removal of antipsychotics. No one was checking what I was saying about the baseline for Alex. Dr B said she had no idea that Alex had to be given a sedative on the previous Friday when they thought he was ready for discharge, illustrating delayed communication within the hospital. The Monday breakage was part of a creative notion that he was making a movie.

Nurses' notes for 15 January included a provisional diagnosis of bipolar disorder as they were now listening to my report of the weekend and seeing the manic symptoms. Alex could not be resumed on clozapine without what they call a work up, involving a gradual increase in dose over a couple of months with the necessary testing, before the maximum chosen dose can be used. Dr B judged they did not have time while Alex was so mentally ill so they put him on olanzapine, an antipsychotic shown to be less effective than clozapine for him when Alex was in his teens. It had also not helped in 2007 when he was unstable.

16 January: Alex's own lawyer appeared before the Magistrate, seeking adjournment to allow time, for an independent psychological assessment in order to apply for a section 334 of the Crimes Act. This section allows for a judgement of mental impairment preventing full participation in proceedings. This extra time was granted.

19 January: This was the day of consultation with the Sydney dual-disability expert. He advised that the diagnosis of schizophrenia should be under review because of the predominance of manic symptoms with the removal of antipsychotics. He pondered whether bipolar disorder was a better diagnosis, in which case sertraline should be stopped. Sertraline was a bad idea if he were manic, but Dhulwa later also tried sertraline while never acknowledging manic symptoms. The expert said that perhaps the diagnosis should be schizo-affective disorder given the somewhat diagnostic evidence that clozapine plus aripiprazole had been effective. There is a spectrum of conditions recognised in psychiatry from schizophrenia to schizo-affective disorder, hypomania, mania to bipolar disorder which can have switches from depression to mania.

He said the cause of aggression in Alex was unknown and did not give possibilities. There persists a culture in Australia's mental health institutions of assigning undesirable behaviours to non-mental illness conditions called 'behaviours'.

The Sydney dual-disability psychiatrist agreed that olanzapine was a reasonable response to the elevated manic mood but said nothing at this stage about any role aripiprazole might play. He did not note that olanzapine had been less effective than clozapine earlier in Alex's life. None of the doctors seemed to note that Alex's dose of clozapine while in the community was quite low when used with aripiprazole, indicating that aripiprazole must have played an important additional role, even if they could not see it as important in controlling his manic symptoms specifically.

Planning as if he could be discharged

In a subsequent letter to Dr A, the Sydney dual-disability psychiatrist recommended Alex continue antipsychotics and not live with his mother. He made a suggestion that antiadrenergic medication (which lowers blood pressure) be tried for the aggression but this had not been picked up by the hospital. In fact it was not tried until 2020 when in Dhulwa, but to no effect except in the first week. Here is an extract from the Sydney expert's letter in which he notes the behaviours but gave no comparison to Alex's calm behaviours when seen by himself in 2009. In hindsight I can see that the 2018 behaviours he was able to describe were part of the residual mania so this is puzzling.

> When I visited Alex, his speech was a little slurred and his movements a bit unsteady. He looked dishevelled. He was somewhat over-talkative and was interrupted only with a degree of difficulty. He was quite distractible and he could not stay on topic. He took my phone out of my pocket and played with it for a while and talked about phones in general. He had absolutely no insight into the recent onset of illness or legitimacy of his transfer to HDU. I was completely unable to obtain any longer term history from him, especially in order to try and understand the onset of

greatly increased episodes towards his mother in September. He was very keen on the idea of discharge back to live with her.

Meanwhile, I commenced an accommodation search for Alex by visiting a house with a vacancy, but this was immediately prior to travelling to Melbourne to see my dying sister. No contact was made available with the carers associated with this house so I gained no idea about their suitability for Alex. After the November experience I was concerned that the personalities as well as qualifications of the carers should specifically suit Alex. The house itself was a small town-house with small rooms. Alex had said the November house was claustrophobic so he would feel this place was even more so. I was told Alex, a big man, could have the two vacant bedrooms on moving in, the second one being for his art and craft, but he would have to move out of that room if they needed it for another client. This did not sound at all suitable given Alex's likelihood to feel aggrieved if he had to move his things. The field of community housing, and what was possible for group care houses, was unknown territory for me except for the negative November experience and the very brief 2008 experience for respite.

As this house was being run by the same organisation which also ran the employment wing with whom Alex had gained a good reputation as a worker, the organisation expressed initial willingness to take Alex. Once it learned of his emerging aggression it was a different story. The organisation stopped taking my calls and those of the support coordinator. However, the hospital never forgave me for not selecting this housing arrangement. I never found out whether this organisation had the carers for Alex best suited to his complexities.

29 January: Dr C saw fit to harass me with a phone call. I was still in Melbourne waiting to attend my sister's funeral. I was now enemy number one of the hospital for not facilitating a speedy discharge to suit them. Dr C chided me for not accepting the accommodation shown to me despite its limitations for Alex and for not continuing the accommodation search regardless of my family grief, because it is "unethical" to keep Alex in AHMU. I was in a fog of grief but was in sufficient control to tell Dr C they were out of line. The allied health manager scolded me on subsequent occasions.

Hospital refusing to treat better

Dr C spoke of the hospital's urgency to discharge Alex and without a community placement, he would have to go back to live with me. Dr C stated that AMHU was not a suitable place for him: the High Dependency Unit was for acute care only and Alex did not have an acute illness!! Again, I hear the bias against him because of his intellectual disability, viewing his presentation as always the same, with mental illness not being the cause of the symptoms which brought him to hospital. Dr C had been listening to Dr B of course.

Dr C wrote up the conversation as explaining to me that Alex's frustration and distress were secondary to the reasons he was in hospital and they were hoping I could get on the same page with respect to treatment goals. I had disagreed with these views and kept saying that Alex had residual mental illness, pointing out the manic behaviours. I agreed that the environment was inappropriate but I could see that his symptoms were not just a reaction to the environment.

According to Dr C, the Low Dependency Unit was not suitable either, because Alex was too readily upset by the many other patients. Dr C would not acknowledge that olanzapine might not be sufficient. They did not give me information I needed such as how often were they sedating Alex with lorazepam, why was he groggy, had they been using haloperidol in addition to olanzapine. And, were they monitoring his absence seizures? Had they received the historical documents I had sent?

30 January: From Melbourne I spoke with a hospital social worker and attended a teleconference with hospital parties to discuss the issues. The conflict over proceeding with a plan for Alex's treatment, so that he could live in the community, was that the hospital wanted to discharge Alex regardless of his moods and behaviours because it viewed these as outside any mental illness. On the other hand, I was afraid of putting him in the community, for the risks, including the risk of further arrest, until the appropriate diagnosis and appropriate treatment were made. I thought it should be possible to get Alex back to his calm self I had known for the previous nine years. We kept searching for suitable accommodation and suitable support workers. Meanwhile the hospital was still using lorazepam without explanation and made no observations or reports to me on the question of whether olanzapine was inadequate.

The picture regarding resumption of aripiprazole was also unclear. This was not clearly reported to me possibly because the hospital was embarrassed about the mess-up. There is some recording in Alex's hospital notes of resumption by Dr B but also it seems that it was soon withdrawn again (Dr E, May 2018). The patient notes for early January list aripiprazole 15 mg and sertraline 150 mg without clozapine. I noted in my email to the Sydney dual-disability psychiatrist's assistant on 23 March 2018 that I believed Alex was on aripiprazole then.

I certainly never had a clear picture of the medicine changes against observations of moods and behaviours, which would have been valuable to sort out the efficacy of any medication in trying to resume his mental health of only a few months earlier. It was already clear that the hospital omission of aripiprazole was making him worse than he had been at the time of throwing hot oil at me.

We kept trying to set up community living despite the absurdity of it

The hospital allied health manager had said I should ring her on 5 February to work out a way forward. I had asked her during the teleconference from Melbourne whether she was leading the discharge planning, including the housing. She agreed she was the lead, so I rang her expecting to be able to confirm who was doing what and the kind of oversight she was taking. I rang on 5 February at the nominated time only to find that there was no such concept in her plans. She only gave me a few notions about what she thought might need to be put in place (by me?) for a Supported Independent Living (SIL) proposal to NDIA. I detected another example of the health system wanting control and another failure of the health system to work as a team involving the prime carer and the disability sector.

This inability for health and disability sectors to work together after the introduction of the NDIS was further evidenced by the social worker of the hospital ringing Alex's support coordinator to berate him for not yet finding accommodation and telling him he should be working harder. I wrote to her operations manager complaining that this was most inappropriate for a professional in the public system to try to lord it over someone in the private sector and she had put Alex's relationship with his support coordinator at risk. I asked that the social worker communicate through me from then on. I received no reply. I do acknowledge however, that this same social worker was very helpful in having Alex's pension payments restored after the automatic cessation of his pension on being taken for one night to the Alexander Maconochie Centre. I did not know and was not informed that this cessation would occur!

The support coordinator was actually highly conscientious and we had been intensely working through lists of possibilities in the ACT and had begun to look interstate. We also had to find additional professional help such as a Behaviour Support Assessment to make an application to NDIA for what would be a huge increase in funding for Alex, especially if the health sector were to assert that he needed 24/7 care. I now had a post-retirement full-time job in getting a better deal for Alex! Between the meetings, the disability sector paperwork, the necessity to keep correcting the facts and insinuations of the hasty professionals' reports, in seeking external help, and providing emotional support and in-hospital advocacy for Alex, I was on duty or on call seven days per week.

And so, it continued with no progress

Dr D was now replacing Dr B who only took the temporary position at AMHU immediately prior to retirement. Each consultant for that year was brought in for a similar three-month fill-in, so Alex did not have any consistency in his direct care, and concurrently, there was no permanent Director of Psychiatry which meant there was no continuous oversight of the facility. Each new doctor added medication so that by the end of 2018 Alex had quite a soup of medicines. In other words, I had no confidence that satisfactory supervision of diagnosis development and clinical responses for Alex in AHMU was occurring.

The hospital wanted to improve Alex's behaviour by offering rewards such as outings and photography for control of anger (while he was being inadequately treated for his mania). In my view, this was like treating Parkinson's disease by offering such patients rewards for not shaking.

AMHU, especially HDU, was in no way set up for care of someone with an intellectual disability who needed guidance and attention for all personal care as well as clinical care. Austere for low-stimulus, oppressive for staff safety, alien with the worst cases of mental illness (a foreign concept to him) and more. Imagine putting a child in such a place and the reader can begin to understand the lack of suitability for Alex!

The stage was set for Alex's unending suffering.

Chapter 5 Doctors moved on, but Alex was stuck
January – August 2018

2018 proceeded with frustration for all parties as we failed to move forward. The hospital insisted Alex could be discharged even though his moods and behaviours were a concern to everyone else for community living. It was not until the second half of the year that the Adult Mental Health Unit had a permanent Director of Psychiatry who could lead the team of psychiatrists. There were frustrations with the multiple doctors, none capable of grasping the full situation within their short postings. There were additional assault charges – this time from a nurse, but all charges were dismissed in May. Manic symptoms were mostly ignored, and I and the community team were harassed by the hospital over securing housing. There was a lot happening but no advancement was made in Alex's mental health; rather he continued to get worse.

No community accommodation could be found for Alex because:

- few accommodation house set-ups could cope with a person of intellectual disability in combination with mental illness,
- the accommodation organisations recognised that Alex, with his current features, would be a misfit and could upset other residents, and
- failure of the hospital to recognise that Alex's untreated mental illness was the problem, not solely his intellectual disability.

Alex's experience in AMHU

All the while, Alex felt tortured in this environment. He railed against me, blaming me for what was happening. His thoughts ran something like: *Mum had looked after him all his life. She obviously had the power to do mysterious and wonderful things. She must have control. She must have done all this to me and could get me out.* He rang me daily, sometimes several times per day and I tried to see him every day. I was permitted in the HDU ward unless there was an incident judged a risk to visitors. I saw a lot of the operations of HDU and the other clients who were not always friendly while ill.

Alex would vent to me during the visit and get upset when I had to leave. These scenes were written up by nurses as mother triggering Alex's aggression. It was further grist for the claim that I was the problem, not his illness, and reinforced the hospital antagonism towards me. Had these people no children of their own? Did they not realise that as the centre of Alex's world, I was going to be the focus of his most emotionally uncontrolled behaviours?

He was swapped back and forwards between HDU and LDU but he spent most of the time in HDU. They also subjected him to seclusion, sometimes dragged in by security guards and held while he was injected in the buttocks with a sedative. These rooms would consist solely of a mattress on the floor and the duration of stay could vary. If he were lucky, it would only be for two hours. I would not be allowed to visit him while he was in seclusion.

I was not always told of his violent episodes such as when he was so heightened he wanted to steal security passes and climb over the back fence. I have since read in hospital notes how aggressive he could get at this stage while he was so inadequately medicated. I had been told he was ready for discharge!

I kept alerting nurses when I saw manic behaviour and when I saw his petit-mal episodes. They were initially blind to both these kinds of events. Staff did not see the very brief absences and regarded the manic behaviour as part of Alex's usual repertoire of 'behaviours' associated with his intellectual disability. They could not understand the need to listen to me as the person who knew Alex best and who could objectively identify how different Alex was in comparison to when appropriately medicated.

Eventually some of the nurses kept a record of Alex's absences after one day I was able to get the attention of a nurse while Alex was experiencing the absence. He was still on the anticonvulsant valproate, the dosage of which I did not want increased. I wanted them to at least acknowledge that it was not preventing the absences and that Alex might need to see the neurologist. His neurologist (whom he had seen privately in 2017) did visit the hospital, I so I asked for him to see Alex as an inpatient. Why was there no holistic care for Alex if he were to be there long-term?

There was acknowledgement by many in and out of the hospital that it was a bad environment for Alex. It took a long while before this was translated into modifying his environment to reduce the associated harm. This acknowledgement of the environment within the hospital was good but should not have distracted from the more important need, and the pertinent role for clinicians, to better diagnose and better medicate Alex.

Extensive effort on housing

The support coordinator and I spent February 2018 painstakingly working our way through potential community share houses in which Supported Independent Living funds from the NDIS could be used. The support coordinator lined up several inspections, including of a place managed by Community Housing Canberra designed as social housing. I also looked at the private rental sector and what would be involved if I could miraculously privately purchase a home for him – again. I no longer had the earlier townhouse. No suitable accommodation was identified and we were to realise that share housing was not going to work while Alex was as ill as he was, after offers were withdrawn on meeting Alex. He was seen as too loud and volatile. We kept up the search month after month. Initially we had been able to organise leave for Alex to visit some of potential accommodation sites. Those were good days when Alex could come out on leave and be taken back without incident.

We briefly investigated the Specialist Disability Accommodation (SDA) scheme in the NDIS but we found there was nothing happening with this in the ACT at that time. It required developers to pick up the notion as financially worthwhile and it had proved too hard in the ACT. A bit later we found that there was some movement in the ACT for SDA for those with physical disabilities but not for those such as Alex. Availability of land is the biggest impediment for implementation of the NDIA's scheme for SDA in the ACT. All Australia is now talking about the housing crisis[7] and indeed it was readily apparent in 2018 in the ACT regarding public housing, including disability housing.

Search for a support if in the community

We also started the search for a behaviour specialist to write the necessary reports for NDIA's consideration of an application for Alex's Supported Independent Living. Such specialists are in very short supply in ACT. Alex had not been under such a behaviour specialist previously. I asked for a quote from a candidate in Adelaide only to find her ability to understand Alex's history was limited. I did not have sufficient experience to understand what she was planning to do in a report either but it was not explained. This was new subject

---

[7] The crisis is a sustained shortage of housing in general and particularly through a shortage of affordable housing and housing for the marginalised members of society. House prices and rental costs have been increasing steeply. More people are homeless on the streets or sleeping in cars.

matter for me. I was to learn a lot more about the approach from behaviour specialists over the following years. After more months of searching, we engaged a Sydney based organisation, with a staff member routinely visiting Canberra. This did not last but I shall talk more about behaviour specialists later.

I tried in early 2018 to get help from the psychologist who had started with Alex in 2017. He was sympathetic but said he had found it extremely difficult to work with Alex while he was unstable. Once Alex was better, he would happily work with Alex again but, even so, he could only give advice as a consultant. He could not engage in direct behaviour modification so he would not supply the help I needed at this stage.

If Alex were to live in the community, guidance was going to be needed to support staff handling what was really unacknowledged residual mental illness. We asked the hospital for help given their immediate experience of Alex. Rather than being concerned regarding the safety for Alex in the community, I was told that community behaviour guidelines for community carers were not done for inpatients. This response did not inspire confidence that Alex's welfare was the primary consideration, but rather that the service's need to discharge Alex was the primary motivation for the team.

In February, the hospital occupational therapist (OT), a wonderful person and thorough professional, wrote the following, but I do not think other staff absorbed the message.

The OT had to assume that Alex would be discharged without any further treatment and did not touch on diagnoses because that was the medical plan. The accommodation had to suit the inadequately treated Alex. The resultant outline of requirements limited the options in the ACT as follows:

> The history of presentation demonstrated that Alex is unable to share living space with other residents and this can provide a safety risk to both Alex and others.
>
> In order to avoid unpredictable triggers, which result in impulsive and potentially aggressive behaviours, Alex requires control over his environment and a familiar team of support staff with whom he can build a positive relationship.
>
> From a clinical perspective the author fully supports the recommendation that Alex requires a supported accommodation environment in which he is the sole resident deeming it an essential component of a sustainable and successful discharge to community living.

Trying higher up in the system

One of my sons, Ewen, with his wife, wrote to the ACT Chief Psychiatrist outlining our troubles and distress when trying to get help for Alex. There was no direct response. However, the acting Chief Psychiatrist subsequently attended family hospital meetings. By the first week of March, I submitted a formal complaint to the Health Commission about Alex's treatment at the hospital since November 2017. The Public Advocate's office had become aware of Alex and was attending many meetings too. At the same time, I applied to the NDIA for a review of Alex's funding, claiming that it was not in Alex's interests to be left in hospital any longer. It would be better if he were discharged, if the health system were not going to treat him. The hospital kept saying he could be discharged, in denial of any mental illness. The hospital also determined he needed 24/7 community care so the evidence of need had to be substantiated for the NDIA.

Canberra Hospital and Health Services was contacted by the Health Commission about my complaint. I eventually received a high-level reply, but it was full of misinformation, which had presumably, come from hospital staff. It confused current events with my claim of discrimination from November 2017. I prepared a counter document. This was not acknowledged by the signatory or anyone else in administration. By this stage so many other things were taking my attention, I did not pursue this process, also recognising it was *my word against his word* argument in any case. There were some positive adjustments to Alex's care, making more allowances for his intellectual disability. Nonetheless the hospital clinical staff and administration could not do the best for Alex while they were ignoring symptoms and records of symptoms were inaccurate. Truth was important for the best approach and policy for Alex and thus for getting him the treatment he needed.

My prime complaint was that Alex was discriminated against because of his disabilities, which was denied by administration. I countered with the evidence of Dr B's efforts to deny him mental health care on the grounds that he just had chronic behaviour problems. Administration claimed Alex was trapped in an unsuitable environment because I had failed to secure accommodation which was available and suitable. I countered with my explanation of why the January house was unsuitable and explaining the signatory had been misinformed about the supposed other options. He claimed I had ignored advice from the Sydney dual disability expert when administration had read the advice out of context. No one was acknowledging that whatever house might be available, Alex was not ready to move to the community and they had no idea how to treat him.

Further, the administration signatory claimed I had sabotaged a solution through a meeting early in 2018 with a community Supported Independent Living organisation. My recall was that meeting ended with the organisation rejecting further efforts for Alex once they saw Alex's volatility. During the meeting Dr D would not allow time for Alex's lengthy talk. Dr D precipitously finished the meeting without listening to the SIL representative about how the possible option was only theoretical, as the dwelling had not been secured by this SIL organisation. Dr D misunderstood the NDIS/disability sector leading him to criticise Alex's support coordinator. I tried to explain, but any of my explanations about NDIS funding private organisations through the client fell on deaf ears with only the model for the public health sector in their minds.

It continued to be difficult to have a balanced conversation with the hospital. They seemed to minimise the difficulty in finding suitable, safe accommodation for Alex. They offered no practical advice or help to find solutions other than advising me to "make a decision". Alex was on an antipsychotic which was supposed to be sufficient treatment; the rest was just ongoing intellectual disability and the ball was in my court, according to the hospital.

Charges dismissed

Meanwhile, to assist the court processes related to his November charges which was to be brought before a magistrate mid-May, Alex was assessed by a private Clinical Psychologist at the end of March who concluded:

> Even with significant assistance, Mr Cameron is unlikely to be able to follow the course of proceedings, understand the substantial effect of any evidence, or give instructions to his lawyers. He is considered unfit to plead, and due to the lifelong nature of his condition, this is unlikely to change within the next 12-months.

It was a huge relief when the charges were dismissed. However, His Honour did say that any further charges would have to be defended.

At least one doctor I could talk to

A new psychiatric registrar at the hospital, Dr F, would talk with me and was not Alex-blaming. Dr F was helpful over issues including getting further genetic testing undertaken to explore a genetic basis for Alex's intellectual disabilities (Fragile X this time). Fragile X syndrome is so named because it arises from a gene mutation on the X chromosome. It is the most common inherited cause of intellectual disability and therefore was a logical choice to consider first for Alex. Features of autism in Fragile X syndrome include many behaviours of Alex's presentation at this time: perseveration of speech, poor eye contact, social anxiety and aggression, including self-harm such as Alex's hitting the sides of his face. This testing ruled out Fragile X syndrome for Alex but I kept asking for more genetic testing for a rarer possibility.

Dr F also assisted with handling the new script from the neurologist (April). The concern was about contraindications with Alex's conditions and other medications. Dr F helped prepare for a trial community accommodation placement in May. I was sorry when Dr F had to move on. I found the neurologist frustrating because when I asked him personally about interactions of anticonvulsant medication with Alex's psychiatric medication, he said that was a matter for the prescribing psychiatrist. *Could not specialists talk to one another?!*

Failure in the community

The May 2018 trial placement resulted in disaster despite a good start. We identified a potential group house accommodation option in April. An extensive preparation process was deployed to support Alex's proposed transition from AMHU to this accommodation. Over a period of several weeks Alex was supported through a gradual exposure to the house to familiarise him with the surroundings. Alex was introduced to the other residents and workers. There was consultation between the treating team and community service providers to ensure relevant information regarding positive management strategies was communicated to all stakeholders. So many people wanted it to succeed.

This community trial commenced very well on a Thursday evening. Alex was managing so well the next day that he impressed Dr F, by speaking on the phone in a very practical and controlled manner. Unfortunately, Alex had to be told he could not stay at this particular house after it was clear he was too loud and incompatible with an existing resident. With this anxiety and a slight deviation from routine administration of his medicines on Sunday morning Alex was unable to control his impulsive behaviour. His mood escalated to the point of aggression and some violence such as breaking a plastic kitchen bin. Alex was returned to AMHU in a highly agitated state by the police. It was a disastrous Mother's Day 13 May 2018. The organisation was willing to look for another house but we had confirmed that Alex was going to have a problem in the shared parts of any house, particularly the kitchen.

Some ideas but no real help

As already indicated, there was a parade of different psychiatrists for Alex at AHMU after the departure of Dr B, whose actions were detrimental. Dr D took over from January to March 2018 but he seemed irritated at meetings as reported above, and showed little patience with Alex and misunderstanding of the disability sector.

Dr E, consultant from April to 18 July, was always asking me what I wanted him to say or do differently from what he was doing. Perhaps he wanted me to put forward ideas that he could knock down. He supplied a diagnosis statement to be used in NDIS documentation and elsewhere, mentioning autism, which had been specifically excluded in Alex's childhood, but did not mention mania. He named schizophrenia without qualification where he could have made reference to the Sydney dual-disability psychiatrist talking about mania and schizo-affective disorder. There was always lots of documentation from Alex's earlier history using schizophrenia only, while seeking to use the recognised indication associated with the supply of the antipsychotics. Nonetheless, there was also mention in earlier documentation of schizoaffective disorder. Dr E was helpful, however, in responding to me about an email query whereas most doctors ignored me.

Dr G acting Director of Psychiatry, acknowledging on 4 June that Alex might be better diagnosed with schizoaffective disorder with depression spells and mania or hypomania, and with impulsive states and high arousal. At a family meeting on 28 June, which was also attended by the acting Chief Psychiatrist, Dr G expressed his views on medication and desire for a transfer of Alex to a secure facility. Alex was unpredictable and explosive. Dr G wished to alter medication by adding Acuphase clopixol a typical antipsychotic, reducing sertraline (tried as treatment for OCD), removing risperidone because it was not working (but it was unclear which symptoms they were monitoring). He wanted to include haloperidol as PRN (medication required as circumstances arise), as well as mentioning lithium as if thinking of mania.

He believed Alex was too unstable to be discharged to the community as opposed to everyone else wanting to be rid of him quickly. But, why was he not waiting until medication to specifically treat the mania was tried before contemplating the nature of discharge or transfer? He was approaching forensic facilities to hospitalise Alex – Sydney or Dhulwa. Neither was possible at that stage. Dhulwa flatly refused and there was a lengthy process to make a referral and get acceptance at the Sydney equivalent. The Chief Psychiatrist's office would liaise. Dr G's insights into Alex's diagnoses were not carried further.

Both these forensic facilities were painted as having good rehabilitation arms to their treatment strategies as well as being secure for someone as aggressive as Alex. Nonetheless, it was a threatening idea to be indefinitely placed among those in the forensic system and quite a move away from thinking Alex could be discharged into the community. I was naïve about these facilities but would learn more about Dhulwa than I ever wanted. Sydney was still discussed in July but then the idea faded when negative or no responses were given by Sydney.

At this same meeting on 28 June, Dr E started his contribution as usual with "what do you want from me, what would you have me say?" He described Alex as stable for the previous 2-3 months, which was hardly consistent with other reports! He concerned me with his negativity, however, about resuming clozapine, saying Alex was on this medication when he showed "these episodes", equating current behaviour with what happened in 2017. He said in any case they could not start clozapine because of Alex's objection to the required blood tests. I could see lack of cooperation as a further sign of his current mental illness and that he was so ill he was preventing better treatment options.

When Alex had been well maintained in the community, he complied with all such tests. I had been able to shift to Alex getting to the pathology clinic by himself. He would keep to such requirements because that was his routine when he lived with me.

Dr H, next acting Director of Psychiatry, met with me on 23 July to explain his ideas. He thought OCD treatment with antidepressants (yet again) was important and he introduced clomipramine. He said he would engage a forensic psychologist via the acting Chief Psychiatrist (first raised 19 July). We should continue with the private behaviour specialist we were engaging in preparation for Alex's discharge. He was very interested in resuming clozapine for Alex. So, was a transfer to any secure mental health facility now not a real possibility and were we back to pressure to find community accommodation? The shifting sands meant no firm plans could be developed.

I only had contact with Dr I consulting psychiatrist for Alex for one week in August through a single telephone call. He reported that the Fragile X tests were negative and we discussed what else might be investigated as there could be several identifiable mutations associated with intellectual disabilities. He told me Alex's dental appointment had to be postponed as they could not give him leave. We discussed how Alex had been well for a long period prior to hospitalisation and now might be undertreated. He was interested in the potential for clozapine to be better than olanzapine. He did not think that Alex should be continued routinely on benzodiazepam-like sedatives. He informed me about the imminent arrival of Dr J who had forensic psychiatry experience.

Dr J, the new permanent Director of Psychiatry arrived in August. There were two other registrars supporting Dr J's direct role with Alex. The second of these two later wrote a poor report for the February 2019 Tribunal Hearing with inaccuracies and bias, but was very useful in progressing investigation of the possible genetic origins of Alex's neurological differences.

By early August we were investigating community places in NSW which had been described as having experience with complex cases and could be made secure or highly restrictive for Alex's and public safety. Places in Hurstville, Orange and Dubbo were identified. It seemed they had arrangements with clinical teams which sounded an advantage. The Dubbo organisation was promising and even sent a team to Canberra for an assessment of Alex. Consistent with many other false starts, the organisation eventually stopped taking our calls for reasons unknown.

Alex not in the best place

For the first time Alex had a birthday in hospital when he turned 36 on 14 August 2018. I had an enjoyable time with him in which he was able to put on some Michael Jackson music videos on the hospital screen and do lots of laughing. He was in a great mood which was fine for a birthday except that I could see it was still unusual for him to be so talkative and excited about the music. His listening to this favourite music was usually quietly undertaken. I interpreted the mood and behaviour as signs of mania. His reported sleep problems were consistent with this.

I never heard anything more about the proposed forensic psychologist as promised to give advice to staff within AMHU for handling Alex in the hospital and for any transition to community. There was going to be total reliance on the behaviour specialist I was engaging for Alex.

Alex's emerging physical health problems included weight gain from the poor hospital food, including *ad libitum* biscuits and no exercise. The meals were often sloppy mashed potatoes with either a piece of crumbed fish or slice of roast meat. When I asked why no vegetables were being served, I was told that Alex had not been submitting his meal orders so they just gave him whatever they could from the extras. Here was another example of how his cognitive problems and habits were not catered for. Alex could not work to the timetable for meal order submissions as he did not know how to follow the clock within his habits! I suggested they just add some salad serves to their extras or in filling in an order for him because he loves salads. Why did no one care?

There was a courtyard attached to HDU but it took only a few seconds to walk around it. Efforts to take a ball out for soccer play were few and far between. Alex tried to make the most of forays into this courtyard, sometimes with the intention of working out an escape. Once he climbed a steep garden bed near a back gate and brought his head up in the path of a heavy metal fixture. He suffered quite a gash in his upper forehead and the injury left a scar. A handful of leave outings with Alex's support worker did include walks and rambles.

Unfortunately, outings were curtailed after Alex sped off on return to the hospital one day. He walked several kilometres to get home where the police caught up with him. A nurse kept me on the phone trying to make sure I did not open the door. Alex kept remembering this adventure and the feeling of being kept out of his own home. It was one of the worst days of my life. "You would not open the door and those police tricked me to get in their van", he remembered with high bewilderment and distress.

Alex was putting on some weight in the previous year but this accelerated in hospital. One of the benefits of using aripiprazole in combination with clozapine was that the dose of clozapine could be kept low. Low clozapine meant that he did not have the carbohydrate cravings usually associated with this medication.

Alex had already experienced a bout of cellulitis in 2014. This had exacerbated fluid collection in his legs from incompetent veins. The current hospital admission interrupted the treatment I was seeking for his veins. It was extremely difficult to get any attention to this while Alex was at AMHU. His feet required regular attention from a podiatrist or someone else who could check for fungal infections. I could not achieve this attention either, although I did investigate a private podiatrist who might do hospital visits. Acute issues got in the way.

There was no list of rules given out. You had to guess about phones and personal items. I had to keep asking, to learn belatedly, that dental floss was not allowed because it was a potential ligature. I had to ask if Alex could be given small lengths and be supervised so that he cleaned his teeth properly. I was told, "Maybe". I got the impression that the nurses had never learnt anything about dental hygiene.

Alex had been most conscientious until now about his teeth. He had used an electric toothbrush too when at home but that was not allowed unless the charging was done by the nurse, if at all. Alex was not going to allow this (his protection of his possessions as was evident in childhood will come up many times) and never understood why he could not plug things into the power points in his room. As described earlier, Alex's teeth were at extra risk because of the two jaw operations in his late teens and early twenties to rectify an inability for his upper and lower molars to meet for chewing. The functionality was not ideal, nerves were dying and some teeth were getting loose and he tended to still use his incisors for chewing.

Another rule was that patients should clean their own sheets and towels. Alex showed some interest in washing his clothes but not in changing his bed linen and towel. No one cared about the resultant hygiene issues.

No belts on trousers were permitted, so what he was wearing fell down and with no shoe laces permitted he went barefoot or was given tape to keep shoes temporarily on. Alex had his own obsessions about clothing and footwear too. With continuous weight gain and restrictions on style the issue of getting him appropriate shoes and trousers persisted for years, especially with his swollen legs and feet. One had to be careful not to bring plastic bags or foil wrapping, neither of which were permitted.

His *petit mal* seizures were never properly treated. I stopped talking about it while I held the hope that when Alex was discharged, we could get him to a better neurologist and have circumstances where his psychiatrist talks to his neurologist.

Thus, there was nothing good happening for Alex. His mental health was worse. He was at risk of developing chronic diseases. He was also lonely and showing signs of depression which was unlike him. Family was very important to him and he was upset at not being able to attend funerals: his aunt's in January and his grandmother's in June. His three brothers were a constant topic of conversation. Now he called them "Bros". He would often go through a list of aunts, uncles and cousins that he wanted contact with. "I just want to go home" he repeatedly begged me.

I was looking forward to meeting Dr J. I kept thinking, naively, that someone will be able to recognise what was obvious about Alex's under-medication and be able to overcome the obstacles to returning to his pre-admission mental health.

Chapter 6 Too hard so just increase restriction

August 2018 – January 2019

Three days after Alex's thirty-sixth birthday he was taken to the Intensive Care Unit at Canberra Hospital with pneumonia and cellulitis with septicaemia. Nobody in the HDU had suspected he was so ill until he could not get out of bed that day. There was an earlier investigation into the state of Alex's legs by a doctor when Alex was in LDU not long before this. The doctor said they were interested in whether the red marks were a current infection. I told her about his previous cellulitis and how it left red and purple marks in his lower legs but I was happy for them to do tests. I can only presume that the tests were done but I was not told about them. Alex did not show his legs to anyone in HDU and no one asked if they could check. The transfer to the Intensive Care Unit (ICU) on 17 August took everyone by surprise as he seemed well the day before.

One of his nurses commented about potential routes of infection saying his sheets were "putrid!" *Yes, on your watch in a so-called hospital where no one took responsibility for hygiene!* I fumed privately. I said tinea (a common fungal infection) between the toes is a likely entry point and was one of the reasons I had wanted Alex's feet inspected – by a podiatrist if not the nurses. The nurses were not allowed to touch the mental health patients. No care of feet, including no cutting of nails, occurred. I was also interested when I saw Alex's legs in ICU in what appeared to be an ulcer on his shin of the worse leg. I did not know whether this was a development because of the infection or it was an earlier compromise of the skin giving rise to the infection.

Alex kept repeating his version of events relating to this ulcer. He seemed to have a hallucination that someone had stabbed him in the leg causing the infection. He would not budge for the rest of his life from declaring this had actually happened. He might have experienced delirium with the infection.

Alex had to have one of the infected legs debrided in order to treat the quite serious disease. Also, when I queried one day why the redness was spreading up to his abdomen, they realised he was showing a hypersensitivity reaction to penicillin. The rash cleared when they changed antibiotics. Once he was recovering, he was transferred to the Infectious Diseases ward (3-10 September). In this ward the rooms are paired for some services such as sharing a personal protective equipment discard bin. The patient in the twinned room had *Clostridium difficile,* a serious bowel infection, mostly hospital acquired by patients on antibiotics.

Agreement to have Alex at home again

Alex was well enough to express his feelings about being out of AMHU and how much he hated the idea of returning. He was not popular in the medical ward having created situations for which the unprepared nurses called Code Blacks to control him. I was upset about how much worse his mental health was. I had meetings with doctors together from infectious disease and AMHU. By 10 September I confirmed via Dr J that AMHU was not able to help Alex any further. I therefore would take the risk of having Alex at home with me again, provided I could put in place support workers for most of the day. Of value in being able to achieve this was the work we had done recently with Alex's Planner at NDIA about his dire circumstances. There were to be visits from nurses to change his dressings.

The Tribunal had just renewed Alex's Treatment Order (6 September, for one month) but with doctors' agreement, I could care for Alex at home. All parties agreed a return to AMHU would be further detrimental to Alex's mental and physical health. It was acknowledged by me, the support coordinator and the AMHU Treating Team that Alex being home with me was not a sustainable long-term option. In the event it did not last very long at all! I brought Alex back to the Emergency Department on 16 September with vomiting, fever and diarrhoea. He was diagnosed with a bowel infection with *Clostridium difficile*! After three days he could be discharged again with a continuance of the special antibiotics at home. I did not have time to urge the ward to review its infection control such as asking cleaning staff not to punch down the disposed PPE in the shared bin and then proceed to the next room with the same gloves on.

Alex had access to his computer at home at this time and typed the meaning of the slur *spastic* which he had heard, or persistently thought that he heard, being used towards himself. He knew the value of a dictionary meaning:

> *The Word <u>Spastic</u> Means: Someone With Cerebral Palsy, Someone not being Able to Stand up, and related to or affected by Muscle Spasm, and These persons Who really say it to someone is being very Offensive, and should not say it at all to Anyone at all,*

Alex managed out of hospital in his own community some days, but he was up and down. Compared to later situations in the community he was remarkably well behaved. He was able to use a bank withdrawal machine and able to visit the dentist. He was seen by the community Psychiatrist Dr A. However, it did not last much longer and he was returned to hospital by 3 October. I had to admit defeat with Alex's high volatility. With a roster set up for support workers, it was an easy step for these workers to switch to visiting him in hospital. This was seen as good preparation for Alex to get to know these workers as the ones he would spend time with on a more sustained discharge. There was a renewed effort to find a community dwelling away from Mum's home.

Alex developed wild ideas in this period about how he could control the world and stop people overpopulating the earth. These were not his usual preoccupations. He was getting more delusional, erratic in language and intent to fire back at his supposed enemies. Staff just laughed off his talk as part of his cognitive problems, not as manic symptoms.

> *Right you all Spastics and Retards Cause you are all These Words Back to you, Because I'm The Only One President James Smith for this Whole entire Planet Earth, I Own this Planet, From Me To All, of us Living Persons*

Back in the dreaded hospital

The hospital tried to place Alex in LDU but on finding difficulties and being reluctant to place him again in HDU, Dr J organised for Alex to be housed for an extended period in the seclusion area on 25 October. Mostly they were able to keep this exclusively for Alex at that time. As I noted earlier these rooms were basic with only a mattress on the floor. They did have ensuite bathrooms. He was assigned two nurses and a security guard all the time. One of the nurses could be relieved by a disability support worker being present.

Throughout November Alex's agitation varied. When I saw him, it was clear he was manic. When he was not sedated, he would go into play acting as a radio announcer and for movie making. There was a small courtyard he could use which gave him opportunities for some fresh air. He would also use it to pretend to interview the Prime Minister. The support workers and I were not always allowed to see him. He could talk with me for hour-long calls. Alex kept complaining I was not doing enough, as of course most of what I did was obscure to him.

The hospital was trying by now to adjust to Alex's special needs, to the extent that they tried to only roster nurses who had shown they had gained his trust. The ones with children of their own were most likely to be able to get on with Alex. Once when I was visiting, I witnessed Alex emphatically ordering a nurse to keep away from him. I suspected this nurse had not gained his trust and had on the contrary, antagonised him. This nurse had previously behaved in my presence in such a way that I got the impression he was aggressive back to Alex. Once when I visited Alex in the other part of the ward and Alex got upset at my leaving, this nurse had brushed past me saying "I am trained for this, I can take care of this". The nurse had the body language of someone about to enter a boxing ring.

Non-clinical efforts

There was concurrent activity behind the scenes:

- Tribunal hearings in relation to a Psychiatric Treatment Order (PTO) for Alex
- Dr J's new multi-agency task force to find answers for Alex's future
- The behaviour specialist undertaking an assessment and preparation of a report

The relationship with the Psychiatric Tribunal was fraught at times. The six months PTO granted in July was due for review on 6 September. An order was made at this hearing for one month only, instead of the usual six months, because there was a mix-up at AMHU about reports and attendance. Dr J, newly arrived from Victoria, was not properly briefed and made a late call into the hearing. Once connected he did not seem to understand the authority of the President of the Tribunal. The President was not pleased and said she wanted more details about what care Alex was actually receiving at AMHU, giving them a month to prepare better. I wrote to the Tribunal and the hospital with my criticisms of what had been written to the Tribunal on 4 September. I regarded the report for Dr J's signature as poorly prepared. I did not flinch from pointing out that AMHU had spent nine months with Alex as a patient during which time his condition worsened.

The next hearing was scheduled for 2 October. Because Alex was in the community at that time, Dr A was required to write the doctor's report to the Tribunal. With this report only supplied to me just before the hearing I found out late how ignorant Dr A really was about Alex even after years of seeing him. Dr A did not recommend that Alex be placed on a PTO. He said that Alex had the capacity to make decisions about his treatment and care! Which Alex did he know? He further stated that a significant portion of Alex's problems related to his intellectual disability, poor frustration tolerance and features of autism, none of which is amenable to treatment with medication. Therefore, he said in his document that Alex can be supported without a PTO. He did not attend the hearing.

I do not know how we had shifted from the Chief Psychiatrist at the Sydney Children's Hospital saying Alex definitely had a mental illness with normal intelligence to an ACT psychiatrist twenty years later saying there was no mental illness with only intellectual disability as his problem. This seemed a ridiculous leap notwithstanding neurological degeneration possibilities in the intervening years.

I had to think quickly and argue against Alex's doctor's report to the Tribunal. I did not really want Alex on a PTO but I knew that without it we would not be able to insist on getting Alex help (such as it was). Without a PTO, the Mental Health Act can be used to restrain a patient but only if it could be shown at the time of seeking help that they are a danger to themselves or to others. Previous experience had shown me that ambulance and others did not regard manic symptoms as sufficient to regard Alex as a risk. A new Order was made until

March 2019. If we had all believed Dr A, Alex would have ended in gaol after a community incident.

Something might be done

Dr J took the initiative and bravely set about trying to overcome administrative blocks by setting up a Multi-Agency Task Force of high-level officers in mid-October. This task force was exclusively for Alex's problems. Dr J emailed me on 26 October very pleased with what he thought would now result in a workable solution. The parties to the task force included NDIA, the ACT Office of Disability, and ACT Housing as well as Health (hospital and community) representatives. NDIA agreed to fund Alex for 24/7 care which we had been struggling to get considered prior to this. The Office of Disability gave assurances they could find funds rather than let funding be a limitation on success. Housing agreed to accept an application from Alex and to consider him as having exceptional circumstances. These were indeed huge steps forward.

We all worked furiously for the next three months. Housing sent a letter accepting Alex's application promising priority for a three-bedroom house, which of course still had to be found. We already had support workers from two organisations in partnership. We found a potential, but not yet completed, house for rent while we waited for public housing. The behaviour specialist's report was being finalised.

Dr J also gave me detailed instructions about how I was to proceed at my end and what liaison would be required. He did not realise the constant team work we already had between the OT at AMHU, the support coordinator, Alex's NDIA Planner and the follow up we intended on service providers, the Behaviour Support recommendations, training of the disability workers, and definitely follow up with the contact we now had at Housing.

Dr J had also said the NDIA promised to help find the right people as service providers. I was never sure what this meant as it is normally the participant (with guardian) and the support coordinator who search and select the service providers. NDIA is the funder. Perhaps NDIA was able to identify suitable service providers from its contacts and experiences but this was not in evidence for Alex.

I was invited to be part of the Multi-Agency Taskforce from 20 December and meetings were to be weekly. The meeting of 20 December was the only time I participated with Ms Katrina Bracher. After that, she was on leave, and when she returned in February 2019, she was in a different job. She said at the end of that meeting that she was pleased I had joined. She admitted she was worried about my presence but was reassured in the event. I never understood what she was worried about. I hoped I was being constructive.

The whole Taskforce eventually fizzled out by the end of 2019 starting with the loss of Ms Bracher as Executive Director and the excellent inaugural Chair. This was followed by the tendency to delegate the meeting to lower and lower status officers. The death knell sounded with Dhulwa taking over the running of these meetings in 2019. Housing lost interest in attending during 2019.

At this time very tentative steps were undertaken for further genetic testing. The registrar assisting Dr J regarding Alex made a referral to the ACT genetics laboratory seeking additional mutation testing following the negative result of the microarray in February. A genetics counsellor rang me on 11 December to ask about the family and why I might want this done. This time the laboratory agreed it would be useful to explore further Alex's intellectual disability. It would have to wait until probably February 2019. I knew that any positive results would not alter his medical treatment but it would help fit together his diverse neurological symptoms which were separated by health administration, not physiology, into mental illness and intellectual disabilities.

Paperwork for guidelines

Meanwhile, the process undertaken by the behaviour specialist to prepare guidelines for caring for Alex living in the accommodation involved interviews with Alex and various people who knew Alex. I was a bit slow to realise what happens with the approach taken by a behaviour specialist. When I saw the draft report, I found out that my honest retelling of some of the recent incidents at home with Alex, while he was ill, was translated into a list of things one should not do in interactions with Alex. It read like a series of criticisms of what mother did as the key to a way forward.

I tried to understand the purpose of this report writing based on taking Alex's current behaviours as permanent. They give guidance to minimise triggers under the existing circumstances but no therapies. In contrast, my thinking had been always about trying to find out the underlying cause of sudden change to volatility and aggression, and working on backtracking to his better self, either through psychology or medicines.

I had misunderstood that the specialist was not interested in helping diagnose Alex: rather, in dealing with him regardless of the causes and likelihood of recovery. Their analysis presumes that all behaviour presented, ignoring whether due to mental illness, can be seen as having a purpose or function, and therefore can be ameliorated by addressing what the client is trying to achieve. Manic behaviours cannot be managed by this approach.

I had not wanted to trigger Alex and had tried to adjust to his new moods and behaviours but it should not have been expected that I knew exactly how to treat him in his new state. The writer thought it was useful to report that I was fatigued by Alex's aggression and abuse and easily capitulated to give Alex the control he sought. The writer did not acknowledge that, in the middle of any drama, it might be the safest option at this stage of his illness. He named me when quoting inappropriate remarks to Alex as what not to say. I asked the author for a few parts to be softened to leave the lesson about not creating triggers and give mechanisms of calming Alex, but to remove the mother-blaming tone!

Housing

As described, our search for housing went beyond ACT to NSW and there were several discussions with a place in Melbourne. The public housing situation was too difficult with their long waiting list, even for priority housing and Alex had special requirements such as two toilets to cater for decent occupational conditions for support workers. Alex could take ages and/or frequent the toilet often. Nonetheless, in December a potential housing option was mooted by Housing ACT. It was two adjacent apartments to work together for Alex's needs: one for him and the other for his support workers. I went to see these apartments in a block almost completed. Further discussion ensued about the immediate environment. However, Housing communication on the issue faded and then eventually the support coordinator heard months later that Housing did not think it right for Alex after all. We could not rely on Housing ACT.

The hospital at one stage wanted me and my son Clive to move out of our house so that Alex with carers could take the whole house with me out of the way. His flat on its own was not large enough to have carers as well. I did not want to refuse given Alex's circumstances but I put forward questions about how this would work. For example, I asked, "How would I fund the alternative accommodation for me and Clive, who would take responsibility for cleaning the house and would I be allowed to return to pick up something I needed or to attend to the garden?". The idea was dropped.

Once we were able to secure the newly completed ACT private rental house and the support workers with a tentative date for discharge in January, we had to do some quick work to ensure that the behaviour specialist could provide training of the support workers in time. The AMHU Occupational Therapist arranged for a training room on the Canberra Hospital Campus which was a godsend. However, we were entering the holiday period and only managed two training sessions before the discharge.

The Multi-Agency Taskforce enabled a commitment for the ACT mental health outreach service to help with Alex in the community. Previously we had been told they would not have the resources and that Alex did not need any nurses in the community, only support workers. We spent time in December with members of the Assertive Community Outreach Service (ACOS) and discussed a transition to community with AMHU nurses whom Alex had learnt to trust. Everyone was trying to make sure we had crisis management plans in place.

Perhaps a resumption of clozapine

It is likely that Alex's antipsychotic medication never addressed all symptoms. His new aggression events of 2017, and the worsening through his hospital experience, remain unexplained by his clinicians. Clear manic symptoms emerged, regarded as separate from aggression, while Alex was on alternative antipsychotics to clozapine, and even after given clozapine solely. Consideration of the views of the dual disability expert from Sydney to resume the pre-hospital regime seemed to get lost for a while.

However, Dr J thought that Alex could be resumed on clozapine and aripiprazole before discharge if several matters could be worked through. These included C-reactive protein (CRP)[8] levels given Alex's leg infection history, compliance with

---

[8] C-reactive protein CRP, used to check whether clozapine has an unwanted side effect in the liver, is also raised during infections or from inflammation. Alex's CRP stayed high for a while, post-antibiotics for his cellulitis and bowel infection, and doctors were also worried that any renewed infection would increase CRP such that one could not tell the

the work up (blood sampling) and compliance with taking oral medication, and the need eventually to get him out of hospital where compliance might be more of a problem.

This did not alter plans for discharge. The Taskforce met on 20 December, and 9, 16, 23 and 30 January 2019. We had our first clinical-disability combined teams meeting on 17 January. No one was sufficiently worried about residual mental illness symptoms to suggest that Alex could not live in the community yet. Sadly, this approach was sadly repeated again and again. What was I to do? I wanted Alex away from the restrictive environment, for him to feel he could use his own agency, explore interests and make friends, and I wanted better engagement with doctors who had an opportunity to take a broader look at his mental health. I continued to play my role in making the discharge happen despite the uncertainties and risks.

As an aside for the discharge activities, I had another call from ACT Genetics. The plan was to try to review 20,000 genes and would need a comparison of Alex with both parents. They needed photographs of Alex as a child and adult to build the story. I told them that his facial features were altered by his jaw surgery but his teen years showed a marked lower jaw protuberance. I had another call on 11 February seeking more information including records from childhood such as paediatrician reports and anything which could support intellectual disability findings and mental health issues. The

---

difference between infection and clozapine, should the antipsychotic have that side effect. It had not been a problem for Alex while he was treated with clozapine for the many years prior to this, but the rules with clozapine require this caution

fuller story was required to seek approval for the expensive testing.

Dr J then arranged for Alex to be kept separately from all other patients, away from the austere seclusion area – this was a fantastic move. A disused corridor had been refurbished as the vulnerable person's wing. This could be used for pregnant or new mothers for example. Alex was given a nice room and his own small courtyard for exclusive use. Alex was able to have more art materials and music. This was ready in December, and with Ms Bracher's support, we were able to have a family Christmas in this wing with Alex, bringing in his favourite treats. It was not all smooth sailing but at least we had it together.

The promise of discharge and the more pleasant surroundings did not suddenly prevent Alex's aggression. He caused quite a lot of damage to the new quarters. Some nurses in charge were very nervous of him but the nurses with whom he had a relationship were comfortable. I visited often, largely against the preferences of the lead nurses. There was one lead nurse who muttered about me all the time. One day I heard her say, "Is she here again? I will fix this" and stormed down the corridor ready to scold me. Note I could not walk in there without nurse permission in the first place. I just continued to sit quietly outside Alex's room in the corridor as a safety measure. The lead nurse huffed but did not ask me to leave when she could see things were calm.

Plans for the discharge to a house

The behaviour specialist's report, when finally complete in December, was too large and complicated for the support workers who had been getting to know Alex and would continue to work with him in the community house. It gave swathes of theory with a few parts specifically about Alex. I was cross that there was some text with someone else's name, not Alex's, as if the organisation just copied and pasted to produce these reports. I decided it needed a summary and quick guide. The workers needed tools which could be picked up readily. The specialist was running out of time so I drafted something myself using the report, trying to simplify and summarise. It was still inadequate for reference material, and when things did go wrong, we could see that lack of ready materials with Alex-specific strategies and tools and the limited training time had made the job harder.

Similarly, the trainer gave a lot of general information at the training sessions while the workers wanted to know the strategies best used with Alex's quirks. Further, the trainer did not make allowances for English being a second or third language among the workers. He did not check at each session that he was being followed. I gave this feedback but the trainer just said the workers were supposed to have a certain standard of English.

The Support Worker and I had discussions with NDIA about NDIS funding for two workers per shift but it was not in his new Plan. We decided to start at two workers per shift to try to make it work with Alex, worry about the budget later and seek review of the Plan as necessary. We would have evidence from Alex's stay by then to back up any ongoing need for intensive care. We also worked on meal arrangements given Alex could not cook, on medication protocols and communication systems between all the parties.

Preparation of a Multi-Agency Response Guideline for Alex was undertaken between health, police and ambulance. I was kept out of these discussions because they feared I would find it confronting. Meanwhile I tried to organise care that he might need, such as with a neurologist and the dentist. We were still looking at housing options because we needed something more permanent than this immediate option.

Mania precluding success

The SIL organisation had known Alex for a while by this stage and was really committed to making this work. The organisation had taken a risk in renting the house. Although I promised to rectify any damage, it was still a risk for them. ACOS visited daily to ensure Alex was taking his medicine. I had gone to a lot of trouble to make sure he had his things he missed while in hospital, perhaps too much trouble as there were now really too many cupboards full of stuff and too many boxes. This was not suitable for someone manic. The manic symptoms made life impossible for everyone. Alex was keen to be there but he kept wanting to do everything, sleep little and had no tolerance for things not quite working with his camera-computer-music technology which I saw as mania. The less he slept the worse he got. It lasted from 22 - 31 January 2019.

One day in the community house Alex got very upset when a worker wanted to keep company with him but all Alex wanted was to be left alone, probably to sleep. On being urged to talk by the worker, Alex went into a rage. He damaged property and police were called. ACOS attended and a return to hospital was avoided. Everyone wanted a return to hospital as a last resort only. The SIL coordinator was very worried and staff had been spooked.

On the afternoon of Saturday 26 January Alex got very agitated, unreasonable and loud when his VHS/DVD player would not perform as he wished. He would not let others help, neither support workers nor his brother, yet yelled about it not working. He did not damage property but the behaviour was evidence that his behaviour could be impossible to handle. He would not accept advice. On another occasion he panicked when he could not remember where he put his camera away, resulting in his calling the police about a robbery. With worse sleep, including staying up all night on a second occasion in a week and a mere three hours sleep Wednesday night, there followed days of intense difficulty. The result was damage to the home, police call outs and reductions in confidence of staff.

On 31 January the SIL organisation coordinator, Alex's support coordinator, a representative from the Office of Disability and I met with the ACOS team. The doctor leading the team was very concerned about Alex getting close to ACOS staff visiting the house. They noted increases in aggression in the last few days and described Alex as unpredictable. Alex was puzzling this doctor who asked whether they should have weekly meetings with the behaviour specialist. Before we had finished this discussion the SIL coordinator and I were getting calls. There was something happening far more acute and worrying than Alex getting close up for hugs with staff.

Support workers had taken Alex to a shop where he got loud and agitated, wanted to run away, apparently to catch a bus, followed by disorientation about who his support staff were and taking things out of the shop, not to steal, but to assure he could buy later once he could remember his PIN. Support staff were now afraid for the safety of themselves and the public. Police and ambulance were involved and I was asked by phone if I supported the return to hospital. Failure again! I could see that the SIL organisation could not do anymore. Alex could not stay in the community under these circumstances. I understood that the only way the ambulance would take Alex would be under sedation. That meant he had to be taken to the Emergency Department to be monitored while recovering from sedation. I would join him there.

Back to AMHU through ED

Alex was in a bad way when I arrived at the ED. He was petrified by what I soon realised were hallucinations. "My hands, they are growing big! Look at them! Help Mum!!" Staff told me he had been given ketamine as a sedative. I was not happy that Alex had been given this experience on top of everything else. They gave him droperidol as an antidote.

The ACOS lead doctor was called in. He agreed that contacting the Sydney dual-disability psychiatrist at this stage might be helpful. Emergency staff were very thorough, testing any theory that came up. One doctor thought he might have been hallucinating as a result of an infection.

How did things go wrong after all the preparation? The obvious answer was that Alex was too sick but none of the doctors could adequately determine the nature of his illness and consequently, determine the required responses.

Once they were satisfied that he was stable after the sedation, he was returned to the Adult Mental Health Unit, yet again. But he was not going to stay there long. Before the end of February, he was transferred to Dhulwa. Ill Alex was unpredictable so the health system's solution was to add more restrictive practices, not clinical re-assessment.

Chapter 7 Not wanted but not released
2019

The rest of 2019 was spent in shock and increased misery for Alex. I exhibited too much patience in liaising, searching, talking, listening and trying to make Alex's life less horrible. Dhulwa thought that Alex would be an inpatient for months, not years, but they would resume his clozapine in that time. All bad behaviours were interpreted as non-mental illness issues and his frustrations arising from the unsuitability of the Dhulwa environment. I had heard that somewhere before.

Dhulwa kept confounding their bid to discharge him. On the one hand they said he was clinically fit for discharge, having achieved the desired medicine changes with the best antipsychotic. On the other hand, they said he was a high risk that required opportunities for seclusion and highly trained support workers adhering to a theoretical behaviour management plan – the elements of which had not been pinned down. Dhulwa was able to use security guards, who used physical restraint, but this was not possible in community living. There followed a tug of war over Alex's future.

In the lead up to Alex's move to Dhulwa in February 2019, everybody was re-thinking Alex's situation from the Chief Psychiatrist to the hospital Occupational Therapist in AMHU. The behaviour specialist suggested he analyse what happened with the discharge attempt in January to document what could be learnt. I agreed but we did not hear from them again. The Taskforce gathered everyone's ideas for where Alex could be housed while acknowledging he was not ready for the usual community options. The Chief Psychiatrist made general enquires about a Victorian establishment that had experience in the dual disability of mental illness combined with intellectual disability. The Office for Disability sought further input from a Canberra based organisation. The occupational therapist made enquiries about regional NSW and Victorian establishments thought to have the appropriate experience.

NDIA said that money was not the issue at this stage. It would still fund support workers to visit Alex in hospital as part of a transition process. This was later modified but Alex's long-standing pre-hospital support workers were able to visit many times. One stalwart, who genuinely liked Alex and kept coming to the hospitals through the whole ordeal, came with us for the later transition to Victoria. He even sang one of his own beautiful compositions at Alex's memorial service.

I also received another call from ACT Genetics asking for even more background on Alex. They commented that another interview would be needed once they had the relevant committee approvals for the expense. Approval was given and I gave them many of Alex's records.

Dhulwa, the relatively newly established Forensic Mental Health Unit in the ACT, was given prominence in discussions. It was said to be better for Alex than AHMU because:

- it was not an acute unit, so not be frantic like AHMU
- it was not crowded
- client turnover was slower
- in-patient rehabilitation was possible
- Alex could have leave for outings, and
- his community staff could potentially get engaged earlier.

A transition to Dhulwa was supported by the Chief Psychiatrist. I learned later that Dhulwa's hand was forced to take Alex by those in high places. The Unit had rejected him in 2018 and still believed that it was not the right place for him.

Before the move to Dhulwa

Dhulwa was supposed to be temporary, so we needed to look at other options for longer term. I had a detailed phone meeting with the regional NSW organisation that sounded very promising if ever Akex were discharged, with several centres for possible placements. The organisation believed it could handle behaviour management and a return to clozapine. One advantage was its connection with the Sydney dual-disability psychiatrist who already knew Alex. It had a large, internal, behaviour support team and would be able to cover everything from sleep management to social needs.

The loss of interest from Alex's behaviour specialist of 2018 meant we had to search again for this kind of support. I had interviewed someone months earlier who had very impressive experience in the disability field. He was not NDIS-registered for the kind of work we needed but could work as a community occupational therapist if not a behaviour specialist. When I did meet him, he decided that he needed Alex to be stable before he could undertake a program. Of course, the problem was that medicine was never optimised to get Alex "stable".

On 7 February, I was given a mini-tour of Dhulwa by the Deputy Director of Nursing. The institution was determined to treat everyone the same which seemed to be based on an in-built notion that everyone was the same – or could be taught to fit the mould. My tour guide was proud that all staff were trained to give trigger responses, giving consistency to client treatment. This avoided flexibility on individual judgement and use of any variant untested responses. Someone different like Alex was not going to fit where responses were pre-determined. I was not optimistic.

On the positive side, Dhulwa had a gym, basketball hoops and an art therapist. A dental care room was used by a visiting dentist. I said Alex would need specialist dental care so would probably need leave for his dental needs. Strict rules were in place about visiting, including by appointment only, showing identification and leaving bags and phone in a locker in the foyer. Security supervision was employed everywhere, and contact with the patient in the visitor's room was only under escort and nurses' supervision. They tried to remove the gaol feel with attractive paintings on the walls.

I wrote to the then chair of the Taskforce with my concerns about the suitability of Dhulwa for Alex to which the Operations Director, Secure Inpatient, Justice Health Services responded in very reassuring terms. The Operations Director said that staff are empathetic and would be flexible about Alex's fears of the other clients, frequent toileting and obsessions about art materials or other hobbies. She promised disability workers would be able to visit Alex but only in a room without other clients around. She also acknowledged that Dhulwa did not know Alex yet. On arrival Alex would be assessed, starting with a very restricted austere environment of course. *Oh, misery.*

We had another Taskforce meeting on 13 February. There was an apology from Housing. Two psychiatrists from Dhulwa joined the meeting: Dr K and Dr L. Neither was keen on Alex moving to Dhulwa while he had medical uncertainties such as his risk for infection. They were most concerned about the lack of ability at Dhulwa to handle the appropriate clinical responses. They suggested that Alex be recommenced on clozapine whilst at AMHU, keeping him on risperidone for the initial stages of slow introduction of clozapine. They also suggested that aripiprazole could be added later. In practice as it turned out there was huge resistance at Dhulwa to recommence aripiprazole. Meanwhile, the Office for Disability, the AMHU Occupational Therapist and Alex's support coordinator were still trying to work on finding an alternative facility or community accommodation covering dual disability.

A renewed effort to get Alex seen by a vascular surgeon about his legs was promised. It was also identified that more behaviour work was definitely required and better skills required in support workers. Everyone was still assuming that

Alex was difficult because of his cognitive disabilities not his mental illness.

Incarceration in the name of health

Alex was transferred to Dhulwa on 18 February. He went in a car driven by a nurse with whom he got on very well at AMHU. He never forgot that drive and kept revisiting how he should never have got in that car, seeing it as a major step into further deprivation, taking him further and further away from his beloved home and family. He did not settle easily at Dhulwa. A psychiatrist Dr M at Dhulwa noted shortly after the transfer that Alex would not follow direction, and displayed irritability. He was given multiple episodes of seclusion. He was intrusive to other patients, damaged property and attempted to assault staff. They did not know how much was due to psychosis, with responses to internal stimuli, intellectual impairment or autistic traits. His traumas were multiplying.

Dr M noted a history of manic episodes characterised by poor sleep, goal-directed behaviour, increased speech production and grandiosity. This was not translated into any mania-specific or mania targeted treatment beyond thinking about antipsychotics in general. Clozapine was not yet resumed, there still being an unusual troponin level in his blood, meaning the possibility of heart attack had to be explored.

Alex was refusing his medications on several occasions now. He could not see himself as sick and declared that he was not a bad person so did not deserve this punishment. "You should never have done this to me Mum." He kept demanding to be released and when bad behaviours were pointed out to him, he would say he did not mean it. It was true that his aggressiveness to others was mostly bluster, emulating what he had seen in movies. With his big size he could certainly appear very threatening and some of his arm flinging movements connected.

Alex tried to ring me using the Dhulwa phone system, which involved using your PIN and a numeric for the approved person you wanted. As I would discover, a call would cut out after ten minutes and a minimum of twenty minutes was required between calls. No guide was given to me to help Alex with this system which sent him into rages. There was no guide even possible because Dhulwa staff did not know about it. When I asked, I was told they would investigate and then I was promised it would be fixed! Surprise, it was Dhulwa's own immutable inbuilt system.

Alex started to use these phone calls to give me shopping lists: food, including microwave meals, because he could not stand any more hospital food, art materials, books and clothes. I would do weekly or more frequent contactless deliveries to Dhulwa for the duration, even during COVID-19 restrictions.

Community team keeps going

We had tried 25 organisations for accommodation from 2017 to 2019. We kept going for the remainder of 2019, with options disappearing as difficulties arose such as exchange of information about Alex, barriers to identifying what they could offer or deciding that they were not suitable for Alex. ACT Housing said they would stop looking until we could give them a better idea of what to look for. One private organisation in regional NSW remained on our short list. We progressed from a video meeting with Dhulwa staff, plus the Public Advocate's representative and the team on 26 February, to an interview at Dhulwa with Alex, to a decision for them to prepare a quote, then to another meeting on 29 May at which ideas for making it happen were aired. Then, there was no contact, no response to calls, a change of management in July and eventual denial from the new staff involved, which caused us to give up by the end of 2019.

Different support worker organisations with suitable experience were interviewed by me and the support coordinator and a long-established ACT organisation was chosen. The selected organisation was happy to take Alex but did not have the bricks and mortar facility at that stage. They kept up with Alex's situation and were key in a move we made for discharge in 2020.

The behaviour support situation took ages to resolve: the required high skills and limited availability of those with these skills were against us. We kept trying to encourage the really good prospect mentioned earlier to register with NDIA as required but it all fell to nothing. Then we tried interstate behaviour specialists which all failed to produce useable outcomes and it was not until late 2020 that we were able to successfully contract the well-regarded behaviour specialists from Melbourne which then worked with Alex until the end.

Disappointments

Agencies began dropping out of the Multi-Agency Taskforce. First to drop out was the Office of the Chief Psychiatrist, then Housing ACT, then NDIA. The Health Directorate had handed over responsibilities for chairing meetings to Dhulwa. The taskforce meetings became discharge meetings chaired by the

Deputy Director of Nursing. I gradually realised these meetings were not designed to go anywhere. Dhulwa had a culture of holding meetings where attendees can be given a say, notes can be written up, but decisions and a list of action items were non-existent and no progress was made.

The Deputy Director of Nursing had not wanted to listen to the occupational therapist from AMHU about their experiences with Alex nor read the transfer guide they prepared for Dhulwa. There was some competition between the two facilities and Dhulwa thought it was capable without others' input. Nonetheless the Deputy Director of Nursing tried to learn new strategies for someone with both intellectual disabilities and mental illness. She obtained advice from the Sydney dual disability psychiatrist's Canberra Office staff. This person spoke to some of the nurses who gave feedback that they really needed more than the general advice. They wanted Alex-specific strategies. They were learning of his oddities and difficult behaviours but were without appropriate strategies.

Dhulwa applied their Dynamic Appraisal of Situational Aggression (DASA) scoring system to Alex in an effort to discipline him. He would not be considered for use of facilities such as the gym or be taken for walks unless he met a goal using the scores. His chronic illness potential was not considered. They would give him an arbitrary goal of scores of zero or keeping them low for two weeks before an activity could be permitted. It was cruel for someone whose disability included poorer control of emotions, in a facility which was traumatic, to experience such long periods of control. And each failure added to the trauma. It took Dhulwa many months to realise that perhaps they could make the test period shorter.

Advice was sought from the new ACT Senior Practitioner overseeing regulations for restrictive practices. She knew of no other suitable professionals in Canberra for guiding treatment of behaviours such as Alex's. She did emphasise the need for the right people and the capacity building that was required in the ACT. Health was going to follow up on a suggestion that Professor Julian Troller, an academic in the field, could help, but nothing came of that offer.

Alex was able to participate in the next Tribunal hearing held on 28 March. He articulated his complaints: lack of exercise, his need for a free life and his desire not to be left in hospital for the next six months. Six months seemed an excessively long time to him and his stay was eventually over three more years. Refreshingly, the doctor's report for this hearing was a balanced well-constructed report from Dr M. Dr M proved to be a very concerned, empathetic thorough psychiatrist. Dr M was also instrumental in pushing the genetic exome analysis along. This was taking such a long time and it was not until September 2019 that arrangements were settled with blood samples taken from Alex and both parents.

Alex was not given access to a computer for writing so he hand-wrote copiously, mostly letters to his consultant psychiatrist trying to be heard and understood. Here is one of multiple letters, each of which he dated and paginated. This cropped sample text is about telling the doctor his personal story from childhood and wanting discharge. His handwriting was deteriorating.

> part two
>
> 9/4/2019 Alex Camerons Report to Doctor
>
> The year 6 party wasn't even great, it was alright, that day later the friends said why were we told to go outside to me, I told them, my Dad had gone and felt the noise was too loud and went and told them I fell back on myself no more of my primary year 3, I in High school everything changed I'm still waiting for and I want to ask when's my date of discharge they have put me and started to be on new tabs, my medicene I'm or was off, now on some new tabs since 2 weeks and a 1/2 weeks ago, since of a time within April of this year 2019. I've been mostly resting on my bed and also doing my work here with my Faber Castell Coloured tipper's textas and pencils on some paper and then I also had to glue some with my paper to thin cardboard that I stuck on the paper. I really want to be really out of here anymore, it's as if I live here really planning on keeping me here for I really need to be gone, How are you faint Point the I should never of gone right past the custom... some guys I was at a penal went to a delook...

At the multi-agency/discharge meeting of 19 April, only two Dhulwa staff, the OT from AHMU and I attended. The AMHU OT said she had to step back because her time had to be restricted to the main hospital now. She had helped with Alex's transition but had to stop. Numbers attending meetings were going to be low. Apart from discussion about the NSW supposed option and the behaviour specialist that we thought was still viable, Specialist Disability Accommodation (SDA) came up in discussion. I explained how we had researched the ACT situation with SDA and found it to be insufficiently established in ACT, especially for robust builds. Dhulwa also talked about only keeping Alex 3-6 months and then perhaps he could be trialled in the NSW option, though it was still unclear what that was.

Support for Alex while in Dhulwa

I tried to get a channel of communication with Dhulwa staff about Alex's mental and physical health issues and dental problems. I had to ask about Alex wearing his compression wraps for his swollen legs, about how I was to arrange for impressions to be taken for a new night dental splint, whether he was being given a statin and other health matters. I needed to understand what medicine changes they were making and how well he was taking them. I needed to understand what it would mean for Alex to be moved to the rehabilitation area. I wanted to know what tests they were doing and what the results were. Nurses did not like me calling, if I got through to them at all and the doctors certainly avoided emails and phone calls. All my experiences with the hospitals told me I should keep asking.

I continued to have problems getting information from Dhulwa, information which should have been freely made available to me as guardian and with power of attorney over health matters. For carers without these powers, privacy legislation was often used as an excuse for not discussing patients for whom the carers still had responsibilities. The difficulties I had were evidence of an additional culture of not being transparent about the nature of their medical treatments and environmental restrictions, regardless of legislation.

Again, nurses were not supposed to touch patients. Thus, they would not cut nails and would not check his feet for tinea (a common fungal infection), and would not let Alex have clippers to do his own nails. I had to ask nurses to provide me with Alex's clippers once I was in the visitors' room to cut his nails. I had to keep reminding them to get Alex to apply antifungal cream. Dhulwa had a visiting hair dresser but she managed to cut Alex's hair only once or twice during his three-year stay. I kept being told Alex was on the list for next month's visit and then when his hair grew long and unkempt, that the hairdresser was too scared of Alex. Despite the rule about not touching, I witnessed Alex being physically pushed and held by a nurse on the chair in the visitor's room. He did not push back but I thought this was a wrong move from the nurse, teaching Alex that physical control is OK. When he wanted control, he would use his size as a physical threat or assault.

June was spent putting together documentation for NDIA's coming review of Alex's Plan, liaising with potential accommodation facilities, community mental health care, and behaviour specialist possibilities. We documented exact housing requirements for Housing ACT to make a specific search. We needed to reiterate level flooring, a second toilet, a room for potential overnight staff and space for his art and crafts. He could not be placed in a share house and would benefit from wide passage spaces.

Alex's focus was on the imminent re-marriage of his father and what he should wear. In the event, Alex was not permitted to attend the ceremony, but his father and bride visited and they had cake together. Dhulwa reported that the event was destabilising.

In July, Dhulwa was still talking in terms of months leading to discharge. Dhulwa agreed it was not the best place for Alex. I thought it was progress when they moved him to the rehabilitation section which sounded better than the assessment area. The community team did not want to leave any stone unturned in finding somewhere for Alex to go once discharged. We tried some of the same organisations where we had previously made enquiries as well as new organisations. We went through what was involved in securing SDA and the ACT potential. Alex was now seen by those familiar with SDA to be an obvious candidate. Later we were given verbal assurances from NDIA that Alex was eligible. The support coordinator and I conducted some long interviews with organisations showing potential for Supported Independent Living – for example with experience in working closely with a behaviour specialist. Some organisations would have worked well if only we had public housing available, there being very little available for rent or even less owned by care organisations.

The realities of housing for complex cases

On 28 August, a meeting now called a 'Case Meeting' or 'Discharge Meeting', was attended by the Deputy Director of Nursing, the Clinical Nurse Consultant (newly arrived), Dr K, the support coordinator and another person from their organisation, a representative from Housing ACT and me. Dhulwa was firm in their views about the conditions Alex required on discharge. Dhulwa staff decided Alex required a level of care experience in the community not available in the ACT. They did not definitely say such experience had been identified anywhere else so I was not sure whether the experience required was available anywhere. They were still not saying Alex had untreated mental health symptoms. A few meetings further on, Dr K was also adamant that only nurses could take care of Alex. He based this on his reported extensive experience with reliance on the 'disability worker' leading to disastrous results. There was a call for adequate training of workers and a ratio of 2:1 to be funded by the NDIS. November was the nominated discharge target.

NDIA had said that funding for one worker 24/7 would have to be very strongly based on evidence. Two workers 24/7 seemed an impossible objective. When we asked Dhulwa to help with the submission to NDIA for a Plan to include such funding, Dhulwa staff found it extremely difficult to project their hospital experiences into Alex's community living. Dhulwa thought that if the clinical view is that a participant needs two staff 24/7, such a statement was sufficient. NDIA wanted to know what the two staff did and how it was justified that any fewer would not work. When I tried to re-write a draft to set out the arguments and tabulate how two staff were needed, I was told by the Deputy Director of Nursing that they did not need my help because I only wrote things as a Mum. It seemed that academic qualifications and 28 years as a public servant did not count to be at least an additional hand. The

Office for Disability tried to act as liaison between health and the NDIA as it had done with health and housing.

We followed up an SDA development that was now underway in Canberra but for which there was a waiting list. We started an application but ultimately did not submit. The development was in a cul-de-sac with intended disability tenants only, which was perhaps not appropriate for Alex socially and their achievement of robust standard was doubtful.

Dhulwa reluctant to adapt

An Individual Care Plan (ICP) meeting was held at Dhulwa on 2 September. This was the first such meeting to which I was invited and could have been the first one held for Alex since his admission to Dhulwa in February. These Plans were supposed to guide care of the patient. Alex would attend these meetings if his behaviour were not of concern on the day. Staff ran through a long list of items in various categories and asked for Alex's and/or my ideas. It could be about encouraging a better diet or items to be followed up in physical health care. It was a revelation to me at this meeting that Behaviour Management was about control to keep staff safe: it had nothing to do with therapies for patients and was certainly not behaviour support[9] to provide the best environment for good behaviour control. I was to attend several such meetings with little progress from one to the next.

---

[9] See Keith R McVilly Positive behaviour support for people with intellectual disability: evidence-based practice, promoting quality of life The Australian Society for Intellectual Disability – Research into Practice 2002.

Alex kept writing:

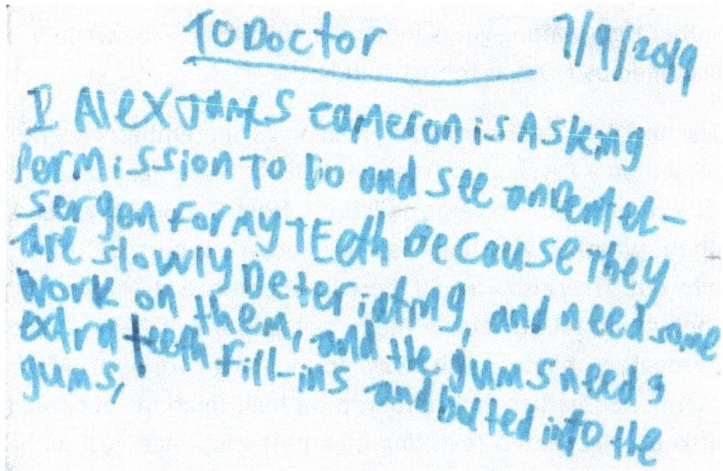

It was reported that Alex had sleepless nights in part due to nightmares. There could have been many emotional upsets he was working through as a result of being locked up and being 'managed'. Later, Dhulwa changed his statin saying they thought rosuvastatin could be causing the nightmare problem. On the phone Alex would talk a lot about what I interpreted was the common subject of the nightmares. He would tell me off over the phone about something I was supposed to have done to him when he was a child as if it really happened. The location for most of these dreams was a house we had earlier lived in for twenty-one years, not his current address.

I was spending a lot of time discussing Alex with promising organisations who were keen to help and re-discussing options with the support coordinator, or the relief coordinator. Strategies for moving forward and pulling everything together to get the funding were required. The SDA process could be a long one and would be important for the option of making modifications to existing stock in Canberra, rather than waiting years for a new build to achieve what was classified by NDIA as robust standard.

The next Tribunal Hearing was held on 23 September. Alex was placed on a Psychiatric Treatment Order (PTO) again but this time there were several questions from Tribunal members about whether Alex had read the doctor's report and if not, why not. They also asked if there was someone at Dhulwa that they could talk to about Alex's perceptions of being called derogatory names. This was an ongoing worry of Alex's mentioned earlier that bordered on hallucinations but could also be a repeated revisiting of a past grievance, just as he would not let go of several fixations that were not based on reality. The answers did not affect the result.

At a meeting between Dhulwa and NDIA held on 9 October, Dhulwa stated that Alex was medically fit for discharge. The stumbling block was suitability of the care in the community. It was the same old story. Whoever was caring for him had to be able to 'manage' the behaviour which was declared not treatable with medication. This was at a time when Dhulwa's emphasis was about the many incidents they experienced with Alex requiring restrictive practices and two nurses at all times. Does this really speak of someone fit for discharge? But they said his mental illness was being treated so he must be discharged! The Deputy Director of Nursing said it was not Dhulwa's job to predict what would happen in the community – and yet she wanted to be in charge of discharge planning.

November arrived but there was no discharge of course. The complexities involved were not appreciated at the time of setting that target date. On 19 November there was a Housing Needs meeting at Dhulwa attended by representatives of Gateway Services which worked for Housing ACT and from Allocations and Tenant Relocations. They confirmed that Alex had been on the Priority Out-of-Turn list for housing for about a year at that stage and was eligible for a 3-bedroom freestanding house. However, no property had become available and future availability could not be predicted. It was noted that Alex had some additional requirements such as the need for two toilets and consistent flooring levels which made it more difficult. Modifications could be considered according to an OT assessment.

We did finally have some contact from the NSW organisation with changed management. They had a robust property but it had only one bathroom. They called for more up to date information on Alex when told why this would not be suitable. The details we had communicated must have been lost.

No satisfactory behaviour specialist

We entered into a farcical situation trying to contract a behaviour specialist at this time. We were trying to make this an urgent engagement given the months required for report writing, assessment and eventual engagement with support workers! It was a providers' market. One organisation from Sydney delayed matters after an initial positive contact in November 2019 by:

- only dealing with a list of queries about their draft Service Agreement one concern at a time taking several days before mutual agreement
- appointing a specialist who could only come to Canberra and Dhulwa on weekends which was not acceptable by Dhulwa for safety reasons and the organisation's Director was warned of this risk
- after a delay, appointing an alternative specialist who wanted her own terms such as deciding to start only after the Agreement was signed, when her organisation had caused the signing delays. They spent only a few hours in Canberra instead of the contracted 2 days, and strangely refused to speak to me even though I knew Alex best.

I decided to cut my losses by the end of January 2020 when all we achieved was the second specialist asking me questions, via email, about Alex, to which she could have found answers in the documentation we had sent the organisation earlier.

The Director of the organisation failed to give his appointed specialist relevant documents, failed to give updates as promised and gave no confidence he was across what his business was doing. This business also had the most hopeless phone system such as redirections taking you to the start. The Director was remarkably cheerful about all my negative feedback and final cutting of the contract! It was all very well for him to say he was glad to learn so they could improve, but yet again Alex was let down. I had to search for a replacement. All the funding from the NDIS is useless if there are no competent providers of services.

Incidental activities

In November the Registrar assisting with Alex had some ideas for improving Alex's taking of medication, including use of liquid forms where possible, a dissolvable statin, using flavours and incorporating Alex's ability to make choices into the routine. This did improve things for a while.

Alex's brother Ewen was married in November 2019 but we never told Alex about it because of the anticipated hurt at missing out on yet another family occasion. We managed to hide the fact that all the family except him attended.

Adds up to nothing

By December we had agreement from the new ACT SIL Support Worker organisation with experience in complex cases to work with Alex, recognising that housing was still the issue and the transition would be fraught. This organisation agreed to search for housing, for rental if necessary. We involved them in meetings and kept the relationship.

Support for Alex from the Office for Disability was now through the Integrated Service Response Program (ISRP) from which we were expecting enhanced strategic support with their close relationship with NDIA and links to Housing ACT, and the community mental health service ACOS.

There was an attempt to resume multiagency/case/discharge meetings on 18 December 2019. It was well attended but not by Housing. The Executive Director of the Office for Disability and an ISRP attended with two from ACOS, the Support Worker organisation, NDIA, Drs L and K and others from

Dhulwa, Alex's support coordinator and me. An update on Alex was that he was doing better with medicine compliance but his 'need' for seclusions was still a problem. Dr K reported Alex was now stabilised on effective doses of clozapine. This was good news because clozapine was essential even if insufficient.

The Executive Director of the Office for Disability made several pertinent remarks about the transition to community after living in such a secure restrictive unit such as Dhulwa, and asked pointed questions such as, "What is the therapeutic purpose of seclusion?" She emphasised the need for a behaviour specialist and a Behaviour Support Plan. There was discussion about a step-down facility as an answer to getting him out of Dhulwa but still with some measure of control. Alex was something of an enigma regarding the cause of his outbursts in that he seemed to be able to calm himself down on occasions but it depended on who was with him. The support coordinator had looked for a step-down facility interstate without result. Dr K thought that the ACT Extended Care Unit would seem like Dhulwa to Alex so would not serve the purpose of being a calming environment.

We seemed to have no roads to follow. There was no input from Housing ACT, no hints at housing availability. The Support Worker organisation was willing to put in a quote but NDIA said it was not even comfortable funding 24/7 1:1, let alone 2:1 (so Dhulwa would not let Alex go). A positive suggestion came from the Executive Director Office for Disability: she could find top up funds for 6 months so that a discharge could happen and talk to Housing. Also, we had a plan for getting a community occupational therapist working with Alex. However, it seemed we were still a long way from resolution of all that needed to be put in place and we were very reliant on getting a Behaviour Support Plan which could take months. As ever, the elephant in the room was that the sub-medicated Alex could not be placed in the community with safety for himself and others under anyone's care.

"You said you were trying to get me out of here. You are obviously not trying hard enough!"

Dhulwa gave me the impression its culture was more one of a gaol than a health facility. Dhulwa was serving a function in keeping its clients/consumers away from the public. There did not seem to be any plans for a way forward with Alex. There were no statements of where it hoped to get Alex, how and by when.

It was now just over two years since we started this horror story and multiple activities creating busy-ness but no real progress had been made. I wrote to the then relevant Minister, Shane Rattenbury seeking help, trying to explain the torment, trying to point out where the system was failing Alex through failing to support those working on his situation. I received no reply before the next election (2020) after which the portfolio went to Emma Davidson, to whom I forwarded my original unanswered letter, and was still waiting for a reply when the government went into caretaker mode and she lost office in the 2024 election.

Those two Ministers were from the Greens Party in a coalition role with the Labour government during this period. I talked in my letter about the inability to move forward including the impasse between NDIA's funding model and Dhulwa's inability to support an argument for more money, even though they and support organisations were insisting on high-level care. I was begging the Ministers to find a way forward.

Chapter 8 Indefinite incarceration
January 2020 - June 2020

I with the community team tried to make sure we did find a way regardless of sufficient help from the agencies. Nothing much could happen in the first two weeks of January 2020 while people took holidays. By February 2020, COVID-19 changed much of the way we could operate. We were determined that planning should not stop and proceeded with video meetings instead of face-to-face. The big effect of the pandemic was my not being able to see Alex in person for long periods. Restrictions of movement affected the lead up to another extensively planned discharge.

I was impressed that the Support Worker organisation submitted their quote to NDIA and had theoretically found accommodation already. I was determined that the pandemic should not keep Alex at Dhulwa unnecessarily.

We had the first Multiagency meeting for the year on 15 January. The ISRP within the Office for Disability was taking a more active role. ISRP wanted a more definitive plan for the transition to community for Alex. ISRP was willing to help Dhulwa grasp better what evidence NDIA needed before approving 2:1 staffing in the community. Dhulwa was insisting that Alex's reduction in incidents since arriving at Dhulwa was due to the increase to two nurses each shift, morning and night. There was talk of additional funding from ISRP but emphasis was still on maximising the NDIS for Alex. The representative from the Public Advocate's Office assigned to Alex's case changed and the new person supported him even after his eventual move to Victoria in 2022. The Public Advocate was ever watchful of Alex's human rights but there were legal mechanisms to apply restrictions.

There was an Individual Care Plan meeting on 22 January. Alex's diet was an issue as there had been some evidence of type II diabetes as well as his obesity and ideas were put forward to cut down sugary drinks such as flavoured milks. I was buying only the occasional sugary carbonated drink. I was supplying most of his food by now and began delivering only no sugar added or sugar-free drinks and foods. His demands for his particular likes were always a problem. There were lots of suggestions about activities for Alex and I thought they could become a reality. Outings, cooking ideas, bike riding, shopping, movies, woodwork? Nothing ever happened because of his moods and behaviours, and then with COVID-19 all ideas for outside Dhulwa were shelved. Later at Dhulwa it was declared he did not have type II diabetes. There was a suggestion that a rocking chair might be helpful for calming Alex. By August, they decided it did not work for him. Dr K reiterated that Alex could be discharged IF he had appropriate support in the community. What was appropriate support according to Dhulwa?

When I noted Alex's moods and mental illness symptoms in early 2020 coincident with a new increase in valproate, I wrote to Dr K on 16 February, indicating my frustrations at being kept out of discussions:

> Please reduce Alex's valproate to early January levels. Given the lack of efficacy, it is not right to keep Alex on a high dose of valproate with a risk of toxic or interfering effects.
>
> You have probably been given the message that I have found Alex's current state of health distressing, finding him suffering so much. Alex is showing (manic) mood lability, grandiose ideas, paranoia, as well as heightened irritability, variable appetite, aggression and night terrors. Mention has been made of his possibly getting excited over a discharge looming. I note rather that his talk and reactions about discharge have been more irritable once the other symptoms emerged. For example, he was much calmer when I first told him about the possibility of going to an apartment, not a house, weeks ago, but recently he has been raging so that people are thinking that is a cause of his deterioration. His heightened anger (about lots of things) is another symptom not a cause.
>
> I have not been getting sufficiently frequent Dhulwa reports, but I gather that Alex's behaviour has been deteriorating since the third week of January. Alex went go-karting on 20/1 and this went well. Despite the talk of further outings at the subsequent Individual Care Plan meeting, no further outings have been undertaken – presumably because his behaviour was a problem, but I was not told. Over the last ten days or so as the symptoms

have worsened, I can see clearly myself that Alex has relapsed.

Alex went to see his neurologist 21/1 and in the next day or so Alex's dose of valproate was increased. Thus, I see a temporal association between the relapse and being on the high dose of valproate. (This parallels my experience in 2017 when Alex's behaviour became unacceptable coincident with an increased dose of valproate, although not to as high a dose as he is on now).

The high dose of valproate is not even working. Increased doses during 2018 in AHMU were not effective either.

I am concerned that Alex's clozapine was increased without blood assay of his clozapine pre-increase. This would have been informative about any increased metabolism of clozapine due to valproate or in any case his idiosyncratic steady state on 250 mg. The urgent need to undertake action, given the severity of Alex's symptoms and the risk that the valproate was too high, appears to be delayed by your protocol to not measure his blood levels of clozapine for at least five days after the increase. The last few days have been shocking. I do not think you should wait for the blood test results anyway given Alex's experiences of petit mal despite the high dose of valproate.

The registrar was unclear about the reason for increasing the clozapine last Tuesday, saying at first it was because of Alex's deterioration and then saying it was part of your plan to remove/reduce chlorpromazine before discharge. If action was being decided to respond to Alex's deterioration it is not clear that the effects of valproate were taken into account.

I did warn you that the neurologist was not going to consider whether the high dose of valproate or any other anticonvulsant was ill advised for someone sensitive to the effective dosage of clozapine: he rather refers such matters to the psychiatrist prescribing clozapine!

There is no need to defer to the neurologist before taking the valproate dosage down again. I note your GP has written a new referral for neurology as the earlier referral had expired. I will consider a different neurologist given the issues, but I think we can afford to wait until Alex is back in the community if that can be achieved soon – to reconsider anticonvulsant therapy. We can revert to valproate as mood stabiliser only for the present.

Dr K did not reply. I struggled to understand what their ideas were. I just wanted a rationale for the treatments in the face of Alex's poor outcomes. Alex would need to move back to tablets from liquid form of medicines for ease of administration in community apparently. Some kind of blood tests were being done. No new leg infection was confirmed.

I kept on the case regarding Alex's everyday care through communications with the Deputy Director of Nursing. Alex's visits to the dentist outside Dhulwa were repeatedly postponed. Alex wanted a watch which was an issue because he had strict ideas about the style and Dhulwa had rules about the watchband. It seemed that the only approved style choice for Alex's preferred watch mechanism was a band made of plastic/rubber to which he was allergic. He kept getting rashes and peeling skin under the watchband. It was thought that if he took it off at night it would limit his reaction but I knew he was too scared to do that. He was always afraid people were going to steal his things so he wanted to keep things close, on his person or in his pockets. I also asked if Alex could go to the Canberra Agricultural Show which was a particular desire of his. He had enjoyed the animals and produce displays since he was a child. It was denied.

Further planning for discharge arrangements

There was an urgent need for a behaviour specialist. The support coordinator found three names to follow up. Two were interested but not immediately available, which was common for this most sought-after profession. The third was an attractive option in that, even though they were based in Queensland, they were already servicing a client at Dhulwa where a staff member recommended them. It was still going to be late February to early March before they could see Alex. We engaged them. They had ideas about how to handle the application for funds from NDIA and already had an understanding of how to approach Dhulwa.

The support coordinator and I met with the Support Worker Organisation on 28 January. This organisation was in discussions with the Integrated Service Response Program in the ACT Office for Disability (ISRP) which increased its confidence that they could make a start, seeking a review in maybe six months. The big difficulty was the start for Alex in the community which would be a sudden change. It was thought that we should use a Change of Circumstance NDIA form at this stage. The Support Worker Organisation had secured a 2-bedroom flat as potentially suitable. This was not ideal but we wanted to make it work: there was no alternative.

I tried to follow up what was happening with the exome analysis with ACT Genetics but could only leave a voice message on 5 February. I heard in March that staff had changed and the pandemic was holding up the analysis of results. Health services seemed to be losing focus on everything else besides COVID-19; Dhulwa seemed to become distant.

On 6 February the support coordinator and I met with ISRP. NDIA was moving Alex as a participant to their Complex Support Needs team which would allow for continuous review and exercise greater flexibility. Dhulwa was reported as trialling 1:1 staffing with Alex during which time they would collect data. Despite finding the two-bedroom apartment, this would only be temporary, and public housing for something more permanent was still required. We thought Housing ACT was still looking even if not communicating. ACOS would not provide the same level of assistance as provided at the last attempt at discharge. They would be on-call for non-compliance issues. Strategies and training from the behaviour specialist were required. The Senior Practitioner (on restrictive practices) was expected at the next (Multiagency) Discharge Meeting.

A meeting with Dhulwa, the support coordinator, Support Worker organisation, with ACOS, behaviour specialist (stand-in) and Public Advocate's Office by phone link was held on 19 February. There was nothing new from Dhulwa: problems not psychiatric, clinically ready for discharge, getting agitated easily with poor sleep, eating and nightmares as part of getting out of a daily rhythm. They were hoping for discharge by end of March. Dhulwa was still unclear about what NDIA wanted and ISRP was offering to help again. What was the back-up plan if 1:1 staffing did not work? Police liaison and having a Multi-Agency Response Plan were mentioned. A Plan B was required but Alex really needed to transition to the community because Dhulwa was a bad environment for him. Dhulwa said it might let potential support workers in the facility to meet Alex before discharge.

Alex's new Plan might have allowed a staffing ratio of 2:1 to start, and with an intention that if all goes well, another client could later share the accommodation, NDIA thought it workable. We also wanted in Alex's new NDIA Plan, funding for dietetics, occupational therapy, podiatry and ongoing behaviour support.

Housing was still looking but discussion with them on the kind of tenancy agreement revealed a difficulty about lease management. I discovered I would not be allowed to be manager of the tenancy under Housing's rules and I was sent investigating possible third-party organisations that would manage Alex's tenancy.

By March I realised that after postponement of the planned February report from the behaviour specialist, the appointed Queensland company was not going to work as promised. The stand-in was now going to be the gatherer of information, coming to Canberra to meet Alex and be the report writer. She was promoted to us by the woman we engaged first as having lots of experience with complex cases, but a quick search on the internet revealed she had only graduated in 2017 and this was her first clinical appointment. Training with both prospective support workers and Dhulwa staff in Positive

Behaviour Support was planned for late March. We requested that this be very specific for Alex, not generic.

In the event, the stand-in merely read text from slides, was generic in her remarks and did not have the depth required. A month later we were still trying to get copies of the training session on video for a wider group to see it and prepare for a question-and-answer session so that carers could work on the Alex specific strategies.

I welcomed news via a teleconference with ISRP in April confirming that the Support Worker organisation had appointed a new specialist to lead the team with Alex. This highly qualified House Leader was a great find and was able to prepare documentation of strategies that would be more helpful than what had come from the Queensland behaviour specialist.

I had a telephone conversation with Alex's neurologist at about this time. He wanted a fairly high dose of valproate still but recommended splitting the dose with tablet in the morning and liquid at night. I do not know that Dhulwa took that advice.

Plans for discharge hijacked

In April we had a rough plan for the transition but realised a barrier was getting leave for Alex from Dhulwa. A great deal of work by various parties went into finding how systems and specialists could be in place for Alex living in the community in the apartment by May. Dhulwa was the difficult party in several ways: no responses on plans put forward, poor communications with us, and it appeared not at all, internally;

and an inability to confirm a discharge date despite the House Leader making repeated requests for responses to the suggested date of 13 May, even though March had been acceptable to Dhulwa earlier.

Dhulwa was also told by police that more caution was required in introducing Alex back into the community. I had no idea about this until the Deputy Director of Nursing informed me of pressure from police.

The police said they wanted a number of trial visits to the apartment over a long period in order to be convinced that Alex could be safe. It did not matter that we had said from the outset that Alex would be confused and want to stay at the apartment once taken there, that it was counterproductive to take this approach. Taking him back to his idea of a hell hole without resistance after a visit is not a test of ability to live in the community. Then there was negotiation over who should take him and bring him back: whether it should be support workers or Dhulwa staff. Support workers in such a role needed funding from the NDIS and the House Leader was worried that it would work against trust building for them to be the ones returning Alex to his detested Dhulwa. I spent my time accessing some second-hand furniture and packing some boxes of his effects for him.

And again, nobody raised anything at this stage about Alex having mental illness symptoms, even while under some medication, separately from his other disabilities. We had all dropped that topic. I just wanted him away from Dhulwa. There could have been an advantage to Dhulwa compared to the Adult Mental Health Unit in being able to provide a consistent consultant psychiatrist, but Dr K never chose to reflect with me any alternatives to a diagnosis or to treatment. He relied on telling me he had vast experience in the field.

Alex started visits to the accommodation while we still had no confirmed discharge date. We pushed on, trying to assess what was working and not working. The Q&A session with the behaviour specialist was held on 7 May with three Support Workers, the House Leader and the Deputy Director of Nursing from Dhulwa. It was a valuable session to have with the theoretical expert conversing with those who had on the ground experience with Alex. The Deputy Director of Nursing finally gave an answer in the negative on discharge on the long-held date of 13 May.

At a Discharge Meeting on 13 May, Dhulwa expressed reservations about Alex having any further leave, let alone discharge. An episode of concern involved other people calling police when Alex was out walking because these people had been upset about Alex using a video camera on people who had not given permission. The House Leader spoke very firmly about all the preparation they had been doing and her confidence they could cope, warranting efforts to remove Alex from Dhulwa. She was very convincing.

The next day 14 May Alex made his third visit to the apartment, this time with his laptop computer present so that he had an activity. This encouraged him to stay in the apartment longer than on previous visits. Nurses kept saying it was time to go, then let Alex stay, doing more with the laptop, increasing in agitation each time he was told time is up. Late in the afternoon Alex decided he would take his walk with his camera. I went with him for a short while, then said I would head off to Dhulwa where I would meet him, hoping that would be an incentive for him to return. I was driving there when I got a call, parked and found out the police had Alex. We thought it was just another hurdle but it emerged that there had been a collapse of the bridge over an exposed ravine.

Just lock him up!

Dr K with the acting Senior Nurse Consultant phoned me on 15 May, initially to give a status report on Alex. Details of Alex's absconding at about 5 pm Thursday 14 May, his trip by ambulance to ED at Woden and subsequent medication and transfer back to Dhulwa at about 1 am Friday, were given. Dr K reported that Alex was still sedated during Friday and was relatively placid at being told that his leave is revoked and his discharge will be substantially delayed. Alex was reported as realising he should not have run away and should have gone back to Dhulwa when his mother left to meet him there.

Dr K commented that he was disappointed with police action, preferring that they bring Alex back in their wagon directly to Dhulwa. Use of the ambulance necessitated sedation and the additional step of a trip to ED to ensure Alex was physically recovered.

Dr K also said he was disappointed that Alex's apartment had been furnished when he thought the idea was to have it empty so as not to encourage Alex to stay. Dr K seemed to be highly aggravated by the whole situation and wanted to dole out blame. For example, Dr K reported he had been told by nurses that Alex saw a bed, thinking that meant he could stay. This was yet another example of the story being skewed with internal mis-communications. I made a file note of my explanations to Dr K at the time:

1. The Support Worker Organisation placed bedroom furniture for their overnight support worker and Alex knew that it was not his bed. The furniture was there from Alex's first visit according to the organisation's needs and was not at my request. I did not think that the support worker bedroom should be targeted as causing further difficulty to getting Alex back to Dhulwa on 14 May.
2. My plan had been to gradually increase Alex's belongings there, trying to strike a balance between making it look like it really would be Alex's home and keeping it incomplete so that Alex would not think everything was ready and demand to stay. At the same time, he needed to have activities as part of the visit as per the planning discussions.
3. I had reported at the discharge meeting in answer to a question from the Deputy Director of Nursing that Alex's bed was still not moved to the apartment in keeping with the view that we needed to wait. I also reported that Alex had asked for his laptop for the Thursday visit and no one had objected.
4. In fact no one from Dhulwa had ever given any feedback on the draft plan from me and the support coordinator for the sequence of visits, in timing or in how the furniture and effects would be gradually moved and the kinds of activities for Alex that would be suitable during visits. So there was no agreement on what the plan would be, but nonetheless, I had been keeping to the ideas of a gradual move with the bed to be left until last and leaving perhaps all the collections of movies, CDs and art materials until

after settlement in the apartment. Dhulwa had been missing in the planning process.
5. For the first visits, Alex had not shown much interest in staying in the empty flat nor much interest in unpacking boxes that had been gradually appearing on subsequent visits, preferring to get out to the lake for photos. Last Thursday he showed more interest in spending time in the apartment because of the laptop and looking in the cupboard for electric leads etc. and said something about the apartment now being his home and how much he wanted to stay.

I expressed the view that it did not make sense to defer discharge on the basis of behaviour related to being returned to Dhulwa after these brief visits, when his behaviour in the community was not otherwise a problem. In response, Dr K said his position is affected by the police view that Alex should never be discharged and should stay at Dhulwa for the rest of his life, with the warning they would shoot Alex if he were brought to their attention in the community. The precise circumstances in which they would shoot him were unclear and it was not reported whether they would use intent to kill. There was no avoiding the fact that firearms are lethal weapons with no way to reasonably ensure their use does not result in death.

There had been precedence for ACT police to shoot someone with mental illness scaring people in the street so naturally I was upset. It seemed that Dr K wanted to stop me from asking what was happening with Alex next. There is a case in the ACT where the person was not killed but disabled for life from the bullet in his spine.

A fight for fairness

On questioning about what it would take for the police to have greater confidence, Dr K said he did not know. He said that the police formed this view after an unnamed acting Director of Psychiatry at AHMU years ago (probably 2018 so perhaps Dr G?) told the police that Alex should never be discharged. The police told Dr K that they would not take account of any more recent opinion and placed an 'objection' with Dhulwa about the plans for discharge.

Several questions remained but the Senior Nurse Consultant said that they would discuss it further with me on 18 May which did not happen. Dr K would consider a way forward given this situation. Dr K had another matter to deal with and finished the call.

I documented questions to be answered

1. What is the totality of evidence that the police force is using? Is a copy of the police lodged 'objection' available for Alex's guardian and other concerned parties?
2. Who was the doctor from AHMU and what was the nature of his remarks to the police, were they verbal or written and to what level in the police were they provided? Who else was given this advice? Is it in the health system records? How long had he known Alex and was it at the time when AHMU negligently took away Alex's antipsychotic medication and failed to properly replace it in the ensuing months, failing to see that Alex was still psychotic.
3. It would seem that Dr K knew of this objection by the police for about a week prior to this phone call and would have been aware of it at the time of the discharge meeting on

13 May. Why was it not reported to the parties trying to consider all the issues for Alex's discharge then – and yet now is being used to deny all leave for Alex and delay discharge? Why does an absconding only, with no threat of harm to anyone, give rise to this? All those working with Alex know how much he hates being at Dhulwa, and how he will take an emotional revolt and like a child will try irrational actions to avoid being there.

Lock downs separate from COVID-19 measures occurred for Alex after he was given a chance to experience a day visit to the potential accommodation site. As a test of how he would behave in the community it was unfair. He did not want to return to Dhulwa, and when he tried to run away, nurses called for police to help get him back. Thereafter, consideration of discharge and any different clinical treatment by Dhulwa to get to a more positive position disappeared. Every discussion about discharge stalled on the question of residual unpredictable risks. By the end of 2020 Alex had spent three years in mental health facilities with worsening mental health concurrent with worsening physical health and much psychological damage.

I tried using Freedom of Information Requests to obtain all copies of communication between the police and Health staff but had limited success. The police department was more forthcoming than Health but I did not find anything very illuminating. I had placating emails about certain information having to be kept away from me because it contained 'personal information'. Whose information was too personal? The authors of these emails? Alex's? I as his guardian should not have had anything about Alex kept from me! Health administration tried to assure me that discharge decisions are not dictated by police. I was given a session with representatives of the unit of police taking particular care in ensuring members of the police force understand mental illness. There did not seem to be equivalent attention to intellectual disability.

Dr K admitted at a later date that he was not supposed to have told me these things about the police.

Nothing seemed to be happening.

Loss of trust

Dhulwa was still missing in action after the visit failure, cancelling a Discharge Meeting but requesting a family meeting 21 May. This meeting was attended by Dr L, Dr K and the Deputy Director of Nursing who seemed to be handing over to a new person. Fortunately, I was allowed to include the representative of the Public Advocate's Office to support me. Dr L had a speech ready, starting with congratulations to all who had to handle the incident, about the complexity of Alex and the need for going slow and steady. Dr L spoke of how Alex could learn to behave with the use of repetitiveness through practice and rehearsal of scenarios. Dhulwa could adapt a forensic model. I tried explaining how we had taken Alex in 2017 to a clinical psychologist because his pathway to learning (in that case to cook!) was unclear, but we had no answers yet. Dr L said in all-knowing tones that 'they' can learn and increase their emotional quotient. Apparently, Dhulwa needed to enrich the 'experiences of transition' which might have meant the envisaged rehearsals of life outside hospital, but this was not explained.

Maybe Dr L was a psychologist as well as a psychiatrist. Thereafter I did not have confidence in Dr L. On the one hand he has said Alex was a case of rare complexity but on the other hand he said Alex could be put in a group to be referred to as 'they'. What was the common profile of the members of this group? How did Dr L know about their learning pathways?

This was the doctor who assessed Alex as not suitable for Dhulwa back in 2018. In his report of the time (only seen by me in the Progress Notes years later) he showed no understanding of Alex's communication shortcomings and had not asked me to be present. He reported a mixed-up story of Alex's living conditions prior to the admission. For example, Dr L wrote that Alex's long-term stay was the supported independent living house where he had stayed two nights in November 2017. He also seemed to think what might have upset Alex was my recent purchase of a new home, which had in reality been eight years earlier in 2010. In another paragraph he firmly stated that Alex wanted only one antipsychotic. Alex did not know what a psychosis was and had no idea what an antipsychotic medicine was. Was Dr L using this as a basis for keeping Alex on one antipsychotic i.e. clozapine only, and not in combination with aripiprazole? I was beginning to think logic was not always applied.

When the Public Advocate representative asked about the danger of Alex's distress increasing with no discharge happening, Dr K said that Alex seemed relieved when told of the discharge cancellation. The Deputy Director of Nursing suggested Alex had experienced separation anxiety with the idea he was being discharged after being in Dhulwa so long where he had made friends with staff. Where did that take us?!! Were they now going to tell me Dhulwa was the best place for him for the rest of his life? Was that further justification for doing nothing and throwing away the key for him never to be discharged?

Despite a lot of talk about Alex absconding and running across a busy road on 14 May at this meeting, any notion of what would happen next was postponed until 3 June. So much was unresolved and soon the Support Worker Organisation had to give a deadline before June because it was paying rent on the apartment and needed to know what to do with the workers it had recruited and introduced to Alex.

If Alex was being treated adequately for all his mental illness symptoms, did that mean Dhulwa was now incarcerating him because of his intellectual disability? Dhulwa was not making sense and its duty of care clearly was not with Alex. I had had enough messing around.

Keeping it alive despite Dhulwa

I submitted another complaint to the Human Rights Commission on 26 May as follows:

> After saying my son Alex Cameron was suited for discharge from December 2019, from which time several external parties worked to put in place the necessary accommodation, behaviour management assessment, and disability supports, Dhulwa has indefinitely delayed discharge. Dhulwa had also been working with ACOS and emergency services. However, Dhulwa has revoked all leave (which might be sensible if he were to be discharged soon) and does not know when it would discharge him. The immediate problem with indefinite delay is that Alex is likely to lose his accommodation, his disability support team and experience more trauma at being kept at Dhulwa. ACOS wanted to see the Plan and they noted the

Multi-Agency Response Guideline (MARG) had yet to be formulated.

The Support Worker service provider has given Dhulwa until 29 May to determine a discharge date or it will withdraw. This spells disaster as it could take months or years to get to this state of readiness again, if ever, given the lack of suitable service providers in ACT.

My complaint relates to the whole government system in which there is no facility for those with dual disability, resulting in my son being misplaced in Dhulwa after being poorly cared for in AHMU. It also means that those who are looking at balancing the risks have an extremely difficult task in taking a client from a secure mental health facility, in which physical force can be used for control, directly to the community in which no physical controls are possible except by police action.

The resultant complete risk aversion by Dhulwa is denying my son his rights to try to now live a normal life. Dhulwa has mismanaged the discharge planning by:

- assigning different staff with variable delegations to the discharge planning at different times. One consequence has been the mistaken indication that 13 May was a viable discharge date to which the Support Worker service provider put considerable resourcing for being ready.
- poor communication: e.g. failure to answer requests for verification about the proposed discharge date until a "discharge meeting" on 13 May. Staff at that meeting denied all knowledge that 13 May might have

been a serious proposal. No information was supplied about the opinion of the police even though attendees were all supposed to be making decisions together. It would have had considerable bearing on decisions to allow Alex on leave before discharge.
- giving no commitment to a shared plan for discharge: providing no response to my earlier attempt to help the process with a suggestion planned slow transition to discharge and no communication of Dhulwa's plan or even if there was one.
- cancelling a discharge meeting in March without warning and without explanation but given the timing, it appeared to be because of the pandemic. No communication of intention to resume meetings was given such that I missed the next one.
- placing heavy reliance on police opinion that Alex was too difficult to handle in the community with the consequence that transition to discharge was conducted with short visits to his new accommodation, creating high risk of failure because of the difficulty in getting him to return to Dhulwa. Earlier views agreed by Dhulwa were that it would set up Alex for failure.
- having no clear idea how Alex will be improved to reduce risk to the public by further staying at Dhulwa except to believe in "re-stabilising" him while saying that his current problem is his intellectual disabilities, and not acknowledging that the Dhulwa systems have not been able to 'stabilise' him to sufficient normality so far. It is absurd to think Dhulwa will now create a state in which he will not find returning to Dhulwa

after leave extremely difficult. Dhulwa denies this is the test and yet it is now being used to delay discharge because police intervention was called on Alex's last leave on which he absconded to avoid returning, escalating concerns. Alex had not threatened the public, was not carrying a weapon, but had charged out through heavy traffic endangering staff trying to protect him.

- having no process to manage the opinions of police based on one temporary doctor's view of two years ago. Clarity about Alex's mental illness versus intellectual disability manifestations is required, such that differences in behaviour due to psychotic symptoms at certain times should be distinguished. Medical advice about effectiveness of pharmaceutical treatments should be provided and a medical opinion about the likelihood of Alex's worst behaviours being exhibited on his current regime should be explained to police. It seems as if police want to condemn Alex to life imprisonment because of the problems when Alex was previously discharged by AMHU without appropriate medication.
- not giving sufficient weight to the torture Alex experiences, the way he has been treated roughly, but then punished severely after learning subsequently to treat others roughly and other ways in which the environment makes him worse.

When the Commission responded, I elected to meet with officials rather than have a repetition of the fruitless back and forth of documents of my previous complaint in 2018. I set out what I wanted from the meeting:

- Better communication, shared planning, recognition of all inputs to decision making
- Commitment to truth
- Transparency on risk assessments, sourcing of inputs and subsequent discharge decisions
- Better discussion of any correlations between effectiveness of medicine administration and behaviours
- Use of advice from the Sydney expert or other specialist in dual disability, noting he has met Alex and consulted on him previously
- Openness to use of external psychologist professional help and training of own staff with Positive Behaviour Support for Alex, rather than Behaviour Management.
- Better engagement with concerned parties on issues in discharge planning with respect to timing and practical matters that a disability support organisation faces.
- Further discussion on alternatives, including interstate, if Dhulwa is too risk averse to consider discharge into the community.
- A strategy for managing the situation should it arise that Alex is sufficiently "stable" but there is no disability service available
In order for Alex to be released and allowed to live in the community.

The Operations Director, Secure Mental Health Inpatient Services and Dr L met with me for two hours. Both were patient in listening to me. I was cynical, thinking they were hoping that if they give me some time then, perhaps I could be gotten rid of faster in the long run. I tried to teach them about Behaviour Support as a therapeutic and preventive approach rather than Behaviour Management which was about staff safety. I was not saying that staff safety was not important but the often-physical restrictive practices of Behaviour Management were counter-productive. I wanted to pin them down to a Positive Behaviour Support Plan and training for all staff.

I wanted the assigned spokesperson from Dhulwa to regularly update me, including on clinical matters. The regular contact was initially successful but whenever I asked clinical questions, I was told it would be put to the doctors, and I never got answers.

It took six versions between July and October to draft what we agreed would resolve my complaint. In the time it took before signing the Conciliation Agreement, I had to concentrate on many other things for Alex. I had to agree to keep the Conciliation Agreement confidential between us. The promises arising from conciliation were gradually forgotten, especially as new staff took over, which was a common occurrence at Dhulwa and to a lesser extent in Health administration. The final agreement was so confidential the message could not be passed on! Any gains I had made through the process were dissipated.

A Discharge Meeting occurring on 3 June was attended by Dhulwa staff: Dr K, Deputy Director of Nursing#2 (new person), a psychiatric registrar and the psychologist, ACOS, the Public Advocate representative, the support coordinator and me. Dr K wanted us to understand what a significant incident it was on 14 May with many police, with the risk Alex posed by heading into peak hour traffic, and involving an ambulance. Dr K spoke of Alex's aggression with staff back at Dhulwa and how they needed a period of stability before we could talk about discharge. He said there was a likelihood of further aggression in the community. He referred to an assessment tool they had used which gave that answer. I had a lot of questions: Why had this not been brought up earlier in discharge planning? When was the assessment done? Why had they been adamant for so long that Alex was ready for discharge? I had to chase answers to these later.

When the Public Advocate representative asked about police readiness for Alex in the community, Dr K was quick to say he did not know. He does not talk to the police. Nonetheless the Deputy Director of Nursing #2 agreed that there was work with police on a Multi-Agency Response Guideline.

Dr K, in a phone call to me with the Team Leader nurse on 12 June, was further critical of the discharge attempt saying he had a letter from the Sydney dual disability psychiatrist saying a single entrance flat was completely inappropriate and Alex needed a secure (community) facility. We had to give up the flat. We had tried to keep the option going by Alex paying his rent for two months after the failed visit The support organisation had done their own risk assessment of the flat and had been willing to trial Alex there. There were obviously different views on how to manage Alex.

We had to chase around to obtain a copy of the letter and find out what sort of facilities the expert doctor was thinking of.

When I received a copy, I also noted he spoke of Alex's high arousal states, reminded Dr K that he had recommended to them that aripiprazole as well as clozapine be reinstated and also suggested propranolol or lithium.

Nearly! We kept getting close to recognising that clozapine was insufficient for Alex's mental illness but on this journey new bends and detours kept appearing. The propranolol was tried (July - October) with initial positive gains but which were only short lived and the lithium was eventually trialled throughout 2021 until the disaster of January 2022. Dr K's argument against use of aripiprazole was that it was old-fashioned thinking and Alex only needed clozapine – an atypical antipsychotic useful for Alex's treatment resistant schizophrenia. And as I mentioned earlier Dr K regarded aripiprazole use in combination with clozapine demonstrably ineffective because that was the regimen when Alex became unstable in 2017. The same argument, if it were valid, should have been applied to clozapine. Why resume that one and not aripiprazole?

The Sydney expert also gave an assessment to Dr K that he thought nurses at Dhulwa were not consistent in the way they related with Alex. I tried to pay attention to this in the coming year but prevention of my visits prevented observations. I knew Alex disliked some staff and made friends with others. He had said that some nurses were mean to him at both Dhulwa and the Adult Mental Health Unit when he was able to be articulate at all in discussions of his violent outbursts. Surprisingly he made friends with some security guards even though they were the ones physically restraining him when he was taken to seclusion. They spoke to him with respect and mateship. There was something about other behaviours from nurses that he saw as being mean. When he was in a heightened state, he thought retaliation was a justified response to those being mean.

I met with police on 15 June accompanied by the Public Advocate representative and the Dhulwa Deputy Director of Nursing #2. Police representatives were anxious to clarify that they do not make decisions about a client's discharge, as I had not been quiet about my concerns. They reported that they provide training in mental health to police members and wanted police to be skilled in difficult situations. They thought the new PACER (Police and Clinician Emergency Response) at which there would be a clinician attending alongside police, would be best for Alex. They also wanted to put in work to reduce Alex's anxiety should police be called to attend by working on a relationship with him. The Public Advocate Representative asked for clarity about whether the current Multi-Agency Response Guideline (MARG) development was for potential outings or discharge as it seemed to be held up somewhere and there was an urgency if this was preventing Alex having outings. Apparently, the delay was with change of staff such as a new Director of the Hospital Emergency Department. Clinical input was required on recommendations for sedation of Alex, for example.

The next day we met with ISRP which was escalating their input because of the concerns over discharge decision making. It was unclear, from what Dhulwa had been saying, what the criteria would be for arriving at a discharge. ISRP had talked about finding some money to keep the Support Worker Organisation involved, as without a discharge date and plan, no NDIS funds could be used for support worker time. There were some possibilities for accommodation still open. We were still looking for a new behaviour specialist. Yes, Alex needed complex care. The Public Advocate representative stated firmly that Alex's current 'food plan debacle' created by Dhulwa was inappropriate as Dhulwa should not be trying to treat his intellectual disability in this way – if that was what Dhulwa thought it was doing.

To explain the food debacle:

Alex was making more and more food demands. The new allied health manager took a different approach to managing Alex by treating him as if her were autistic. If Alex were autistic he was not typically so. Autism had been specifically excluded in his childhood. Dhulwa thought if he could agree to a certain list of breakfast foods, then that is all he would get and he would accept this with no resultant rages. I tried to protest for Alex.

He did not know they wanted a contract. What they did not understand was Alex was not capable of planning like that for a future event in terms of limited kinds of foods and strict numbers of each. He just saw their pictures of foods (they used pictures even though Alex could read quite well) as indicating they would give him lots of these foods. Staff tried to say he had to finish what he had been given already before anything else, either more food on his tray or another activity. Alex just wanted to see the full selection potential set out on his food tray. It was a ritual.

He would often storm to his room without eating, giving up on the dispute. All his incident notes for the period were about food times. He was losing weight, which was a good thing really but it was accompanied by a less nutritional diet. They put him on multivitamin tablets.

The remainder of the year was filled with anxiety and confusion, but also hard work by the team which was trying to resurrect something of a discharge plan. Some very dedicated people held some hope and, concentrating on Alex's human rights, kept pushing forward.

Chapter 9 Despair then remarkable hope
July 2020 - February 2021

Far from showing signs of relief about still being in Dhulwa as reported by Dr K, Alex kept telling me he hated Dhulwa. He would often bellow at me about getting him out. He could not understand why I needed to do so much searching for accommodation when in his mind he could just go home. He was non-compliant with medicines many times. Leg pain was a frequent problem. Staff kept telling me that he could be aggressive and hurt people. I and his community team kept striving but we seemed to be marking time.

Alex would give me shopping lists almost daily. He wanted his constant supply of preferred foods. I could not tell whether he really had run out of items or the nurses were just telling him they were depleted to avoid being asked to serve them again. I know Dhulwa purchased an extra fridge for his food. When I had been allowed to visit pre-COVID I could casually get answers about the stores from the nurses accompanying him to the visitors' room. Now I was in trouble with the lack of contact with Alex because of COVID restrictions and was lectured by a nurse one delivery day about how I was operating contrary to what management wanted. I told her I did not have x-ray vision to know what Alex had in store. They needed to let me know. There were a few nurses who despised me and a few at the opposite end who respected my advocacy for Alex.

He still seemed to be having trouble getting a usable watch and with shaving because he wanted to use an electric shaver. He kept asking for his DS game machine but I had already supplied it to Dhulwa, which never seemed to be able to give me an answer about whether it had been approved or not. Art materials and access to the art room were constantly questioned but not resolved. He went through several (second hand) MD3 players and an iPod while at Dhulwa, having smashed these in frustration over something. Alex certainly let me know of his frustrations over the phone. I was in no doubt that Alex had to be removed from Dhulwa.

In March 2020 I made a submission to the Royal Commission into Violence, Abuse, Neglect and Exploitation of People with Disability which had just opened with the first tranche being an inquiry on the health services domain. I set out my complaints about the insistence that he had behavioural problems not mental illness or that they attributed some mental health symptoms to behaviour due to intellectual disability, about the failure to consult me, his carer, as best substitute for being able to consult Alex and the negligence of physical health matters. I ended the submission with some positivity because Alex had shown improvement and discharge was being discussed again. In the long run of course, this was misplaced. The Commission's report in September 2023 reveals Alex was not alone in suffering diagnostic overshadowing and discrimination by failure to approach him differently in mental illness assessments.

Meanwhile we worked on all the threads hoping to keep discharge alive. There were movements on who was leading discharge, we appointed yet another behaviour specialist, public housing was still open, but Dhulwa was still being difficult.

Alex suffers while administrations flounder

Dhulwa was finding it difficult to clarify their roles and responsibilities with the loss of the Deputy Director of Nursing #1 and its reaction to the failed accommodation visit in May. There were high level talks in June with an escalation within the Integrated Support Program (ISRP) of the Office for Disability. ISRP wanted to take over chairing of 'case meetings', to operate under terms of reference, with follow up of action items. Dhulwa had meetings without objectives. We had several ISRP meetings from July to September but subsequently Dhulwa seemed to be now interested in managing discharge under their new allied health manager. The Dhulwa social worker did search for accommodation for two months, only found negative responses from suppliers and then moved to another position.

Thus the ball was back in the disability court again, but another barrier was that Alex was adamant he did not want to move interstate. Dhulwa did not seem to want to work with the non-health members of the team, implying health facility staff were the only ones who could manage a discharge. I pointed out to Dr K that it was his nurses who were in charge of the failed visit in May, not the House Leader from the Support

Worker organisation who was present for most of the day, but as an observer.

Discussion and agreement were needed at a high administrative level on who was driving and coordinating discharge. However, responsibilities changed again towards the end of the year. The Public Advocate was consulted. ISRP gave me and the support coordinator a handover update on 21 August. After months wanting to get more involved, ISRP made a decision to withdraw at the end of August. Housing Directorate liaison responsibilities would pass to the support coordinator. The behaviour specialist would liaise with the allied health manager to help with communications to Alex while still in Dhulwa as well as discharge. Dhulwa would now coordinate input from all agencies/professionals. Searching for the secure community facilities suggested continued.

Searching for providers again

The support coordinator made enquiries with several accommodation places over June and July. Interstate was going to be very difficult where clients in their own state were already on the waiting lists, if there were ever vacancies at all. The allied health manager persisted with Disability Services Australia as an option. SDA was spoken of more but we would need an application backed up by a behaviour specialist and there was nothing yet in the ACT. Nothing about SDA happened overnight.

We had told the Queensland behaviour specialist organisation of Alex's indefinite discharge delay, and considering the COVID restrictions on travel to and from Queensland, we put their contract into abeyance. This was not done lightly. Everyone was mindful, if we were to move forward to a better discharge plan, that work from a highly qualified behaviour specialist was critical. We tried the one we knew based in Melbourne whom we had asked twice previously. This company had a representative located nearby so did not have a problem with travel restrictions from Melbourne. They now thought they had capacity to work with Alex and we started having them attend our meetings and provided background documents as soon as we could. This was very positive.

Housing ACT was still supposed to be looking. A new representative from Housing came to a Case Meeting on 26 August asking for details of the housing requirements. We asked what happened to the previous reports we had provided months earlier. We said we would be happy to forward the reports again and send the minutes of the meeting with Housing from November 2019, at which we had promises from Housing for Alex on the Out of Turn list. We did not have confidence in Housing ACT.

I undertook further work on the potential lease arrangements in the hope public housing could work. I chased organisations which might take the head lease for a house under public housing. We had reduced the list to one organisation, but different conversations there with different people brought different answers. There also seemed to be a communication breakdown between Housing and this organisation. Why was there not a system which actually worked in this field? Wherever I turned I got blocked. The housing organisation's story seemed confused with their role as a direct provider of accommodation and with no vacancies, the organisation wanted to dispose of my enquiry. I had a video meeting with

Housing on 22 September at which the discussion about a head lease indicated it would all be possible. The difficulties were being able to meet Alex's requirements and managing the lack of a discharge date.

In November, still not certain that my request was understood, the support coordinator and I accepted that the answer from the housing organisation was negative. Someone from Housing ACT was going to speak with Specialty Housing and we all needed to clarify the NDIA position on lease arrangements. On 23 November I had a direct call from the provider saying, it could take a 'head lease' after all, despite previous statements.

There was no accommodation in the offing anyway. Alternatives were still being sought: the support worker organisation was still looking, trying to consider for example new houses, and we discovered SDA in the robust category[10] was possibly starting in ACT. Good news but it would take at least two years, or perhaps longer if planning approvals were a problem.

The 26 August Case Conference was the last being chaired by ISRP. Much was now going to depend on the behaviour specialist for improvements in the way Dhulwa was working with Alex, for supporting discharge, with behaviour planning and training of support workers and for assisting Housing ACT

---

[10] There are several SDA categories not all suitable for Alex. For example, if the dwelling was designed to have a hoist over the bed and wide doorways but not designed with strengthened walls and other robust fittings, it would not be suitable

understand the requirements for Alex. I was despondent as there was no progress.

Frustration with Dhulwa

I experienced another example of the failure of internal communications within Dhulwa in November. Alex had been kept at Dhulwa unable to keep a dentist appointment again. Alex had a broken tooth and others were loose. The Dhulwa visiting dentist had arranged for another night splint but made it for the upper teeth instead of the lower teeth and it was his upper teeth which might have needed crowns. This might have altered splint fit. The allied health manager explained that the Leave Committee had stipulated that Alex was only allowed leave for the dentist if the leave of the previous week to go bush walking was successful. On two occasions they tried the bush walk but the first time he was upset and the second he said he was too tired. No one, certainly not Alex, had intended or realised that missing the bush walk altogether with no test of success as an outing, would mean missing the much-needed dental appointment. The allied health manager apologised for this lack of elementary communication regarding leave. It also spoke to me of Dhulwa's limited idea of how to 'test' Alex.

Alex was quite articulate about his frustrations at Dhulwa at this stage and it was good that the allied health manager stayed in frequent contact. She was able to give me (mostly) more timely responses about what Alex was allowed to have regarding watches and music playing devices etc. One of his complaints was about nurses distracting him, when they wanted something, with threats to go in his room and mess with his things. This was a particular phobia of his and they played on it. They would laugh at him when he panicked, rushing to try to stop them. The allied health manager agreed with me that this was not good professional practice and promised it would stop. I witnessed the trickery myself as still standard practice in 2022 in Dhulwa where Alex was indeed still incarcerated!

On a phone call from the allied health manager and the Clinical Nurse Consultant on 10 July, I was told Alex had been having bad sleep and the previous night he had not slept at all. His irritability was increasing, resulting in him hurting nurses, despite the initial calming effect of propranolol. He was still losing weight. They were having trouble administering medicine. They could not tell what would trigger non-compliance. They were searching for ideas and suggested maybe video calls to me as a reward.

The support coordinator noted to me on 13 July that Dhulwa had the list of what we had tried for accommodation already but nothing more had happened. There was no feedback from Housing ACT. The Dhulwa social worker had made contact with the NSW regional organisation, as we had, but nothing else was happening.

I determined that the risk assessment tool that Dhulwa was using for Alex's risk in the community was the Historical Clinical Risk Management – 20 HCR–20 (Webster, Douglas, Eaves, & Hart, 1997) developed for the assessment of general violence in forensic-psychiatric patients. It uses structured professional judgement decision making, not probabilities against large sampled data. There have been updated versions developed. I have no information about how it was used for Alex, how risk factors were chosen, whether it was from an interview. The behaviour specialist's view when we had appointed one, was that this tool was not suited for those with intellectual disability. She said we needed to use the dynamic factors such as clinical presentation not the static ones such as historic records.

In the lead up to Alex's 38th birthday he was not stable, the meal disciplining was causing upsets and medicine compliance was variable. I was told on 11 August that there were no rules being applied to meals but on 13 August at the Individual Care Plan (ICP) meeting I raised it as a major issue to try to get clarity. Did they think they could discipline him out of his autism? The nurses would try something different by administering some of the medicine early e.g. 6 am before breakfast. The ability to let him into the gym and the art room was compromised because of his aggression. Also in the art room he was interfering with other clients' things in the cupboards. Dr K was worried about Alex's lack of showering. Toileting for hours was another issue. He still had pain in the shin of his left leg. And so we went through the ICP list again.

I took in all the special food with cakes that Alex asked for his birthday on 14 August which we could not have together. He was highly aroused for the next week about getting out. I chased up whether his presents had been given to him but was given only vague answers. Nurses were adopting a line up approach in silence after offering the breakfast items. Alex began referring to how much he hated them standing like "a brick wall". They tried increasing the propranolol and then tried Acuphase to little effect.

A genetic diagnosis

I knew that it was not going to provide a solution for Alex's predicament but at long last there was a genetic finding from the analysis of Alex's results from the genetics laboratory. Whole exome sequencing was performed for Alex and his parents. I was told Dr Freckmann from ACT Genetics would call me on 4 September. I received a copy of the genetics report and was given an opportunity to ask questions of her. Alex was found to have a rare, de novo (not inherited) frameshift mutation at the chromosome location for the protein ASH1L. This meant that he had disruptions in the proper reading of the gene that was important in nerve development. At last, a cause of Alex's multiple neurological problems was found. (see Attachment for more details)

There was a possibility that this was the single cause of all his disabilities intellectual and psychiatric. There are now publications linking mutations at the ASH1L site with a range of neurodegenerative conditions: developmental delay, intellectual disability, autism, schizophrenia, attentional deficit disorder and epilepsy. Other genes affecting nerve development can be linked to these conditions and diseases, presumably because there are multiple steps in the relevant neurological development stages.

Not enough was known about this mutation to be able to predict the progression of Alex's problems, most published studies looking at the most severely intellectually disabled cases. Could Alex's mutation mean his problems were neurodegenerative and worsening? There has not been much published overall on this mutation but it is becoming increasingly significant in explaining phenotypes such as Alex's, beyond being regarded as a peculiar enigma. Because ASH1L has an action which is epigenetic in nature (meaning it affects the way other nerve development genes are expressed) each trajectory for anyone with a mutation at this site could vary. It definitely affects brain development in early life and because of the way nerves continue to grow and re-connect, it could have additional effects as the individual matures and experiences different things in life.

I thought it extremely important for those caring for him to appreciate that it was not his fault. He was not just badly brought up or, in the extreme, an evil person. He was just given a very short straw. It was also important for his doctors and nurses to see a unifying explanation for what was appearing to them as separate illnesses. It should have helped them see that Alex was not going to fit into their typical profiles and a re-think might have been required, or maybe some of the things I had been saying to them would make more sense.

Dr M was back and very interested given their efforts in making sure this genetic testing was done and with their interest in considering Alex broadly, rather than simply someone with maybe schizophrenia plus intellectual disabilities and funny ways. Dr M was sure that there was something deeper to be explored to explain Alex. Translation of this understanding to better medicines for him was not possible, as medication is directed towards the symptoms of genetic expression (the phenotype) only as far as this is interpreted by clinicians. Perhaps his type of schizophrenia or schizoid afferent disorder might have been better understood given the genetic basis for his cluster of symptoms so labelled. I speculated that future research might enable a genetic approach to more appropriate pharmaceutical treatments for individuals.

I wanted everyone to know Alex's fate

The next Tribunal hearing occurred on 7 September. I had written to the President of the Tribunal in June expressing my concerns about the continued placement of Alex in Dhulwa. I understood it is not the role of the Tribunal to recommend a facility for the Treatment Order, or to make comments about how a facility is run. Their Treatment Order legally assigns the patient to the Chief Psychiatrist who then is responsible for how treatment is given and usually means the patient can be involuntarily kept in a facility. The place of care is supposed to be the least restrictive that is necessary. I thought the Tribunal needed to know that Alex was getting worse while at Dhulwa.

Alex had been at Dhulwa nineteen months. I had said in my letter to the President, written when Dhulwa seemed to be never going to discharge Alex:

> However hard Dhulwa has tried, there has been no net improvement in behaviours of concern from the time of admittance in February 2019, except from some reduction in manic and other psychotic symptoms after moving to an effective dose of clozapine. The allied health treatments have been overall ineffective, despite some short periods of calm at times. Nothing is sustained as staff rapidly move on with no continuity in understanding of Alex. For his stabilisation since 14 May, Dhulwa says it is working hard to support him but it does not seem as if there is any

evidence that staff are trying anything new in the last three weeks and his current state is highly volatile. It is a design for failure, as all the environmental and systemic arrangements and approaches ensure Alex does not calm down, defending the Dhulwa argument that he is too great a risk to discharge.

If Dhulwa could acknowledge its shortcomings, it could profitably seek help elsewhere, including letting other professionals work with Alex from outside.

I was pleased to hear that the behaviour specialist's team member available in Canberra planned to visit Alex in Dhulwa to start the process of gathering information for the behaviour assessment. However, it was going to take until the end of January 2021 to produce a Model of Care for Alex while in the community. Concurrently we had many questions to put to the organisation because there seemed to be no answers inside Dhulwa for dealing with his moods, demands and aggression. I knew something of his state from his phone calls and continual obsession about foods, art materials, clothing, wanting more and more layers, potential outings and equipment. At least staff members were able to get him out on their walking track more, congratulating him on record laps. I kept asking for Alex to get a haircut but nothing happened.

Alex having video sessions with me helped his moods. The allied health manager was getting to know him and developed a good relationship with him. She was paying attention to his environment. At this time it was evident to me, nonetheless, that Alex had manic symptoms still. Apart from his sleeplessness and arousal about his possessions, he also asked me for various costume items. These were for pretend scenarios for maybe movies and playacting. For example, he asked for a yellow raincoat so he could be a weird scientist in a basketball movie. My claims that this was not part of Alex's behaviour when he was at a stable baseline were ignored so I just went along with helping any of these ideas. I do not think he ever wore the raincoat.

When the allied health manager finally had contact with the elusive Disability Services Australia (which ordinary people could not contact) she put various questions to them by email. They had experience with challenging behaviours. We submitted a registration form.

Escalation to friction with Dhulwa

It was difficult for Alex's community team to work with Dhulwa. In October Dr K gave another outburst, about no confidence in any disability workers in the ACT and about the difficulties and sometimes assault that the nurses at Dhulwa faced. Dr K seemed to believe that NSW disability workers would be capable but did not explain. He brought up Alex's failed attempt in the community in January 2019 as evidence of the uselessness of the ACT. I heard later that Dr K had experienced some disasters with other patients reliant on disability workers in the community, which could explain his extraordinary claim that support providers wanted to put their staff in danger! Certainly, the existence of the NDIS had prompted many to enter the sector with no watch on qualifications, experience and standards. I understood it was up to me to discriminate among the organisations for experience with complex cases and use recommendations from others. The irony is, as we could see more clearly later, Alex's risks were due to mental illness symptoms that were Dr K's responsibilities.

November came but there was no progress. Dhulwa continued to have trouble recruiting people with the required range of skills. People kept leaving and few were interested in applying for the allied health vacancies. Accurate writing was often compromised.

Accurate documentation in dealing with all the agencies was important. There was a classic case in 2018 where a document approved by the Deputy Director of Nursing said Alex had only two brothers and had a girlfriend at some stage. When I tried to correct these errors and others, I was ignored. Did they think that I did not know how many brothers Alex had? The girlfriend was a fiction created from my comment to the social worker about social contact with some of those previously at Black Mountain School. This group included a female.

The latest problem was an occupational therapy report being prepared for Housing ACT and the next review of Alex's NDIS Plan. The report had errors of fact, such as the wrong age and the invention that Alex had an OT assessment in the community when he had no such assessment. It said he had a routine in Dhulwa and he would not get such good support in the community. I do not know how the chaos he created in Dhulwa was a routine. And the report gave absconding in the community as an example of Alex's violence! There were other misrepresentations of Alex's issues. I emailed the allied health manager with my recommended amendments and corrections of invented ideas. I was always on guard for messaging to be effective and not creating documents that later would be regarded as gospel and perpetuated as fact. After no response for ages, she told me the OT had left.

Alex kept trying politely to do things as part of normal life. In the photograph of another page of his writing it is heartbreaking to see how much he thought of family at Christmas when most contact with those he loved was denied. He begged for leave to buy Christmas presents in this page.

The Dhulwa Christmas party in early December, to which parents may go to share in a lunch, started well. I had a good time with Alex who was restricted to the visitor's room for the party so that any difficulty with other residents would be avoided. He was quiet and well behaved. He got a bit excited when the visiting musician came in and the room was a bit crowded with the nurses, Dr M and another. He at first joined in then seemed overwhelmed but stayed quiet. Nurses edged closer to me with more approaching the room. They had decided it was the end of the visit. I had not. Security guards descended and Alex got upset. They forcibly removed him and put me in the corridor. I lost it. "You did this", I screamed at them. "We were having a good time. You ruined it with your heavy tactics. You just scared Alex unnecessarily." Certain staff came to sit me down and wait for my tears to subside. I was not reassured by Dr L's contribution that Dhulwa knew what they were doing, although I appreciated his coming to see me.

The allied health manager, the support coordinator and I met with Disability Services Australia (DSA) on 17 December. This was useful with lots of questions being answered but there were no options immediately suitable and available. The allied health manager asked several questions about the availability of nursing services in the houses – emphasising that this was something the Dhulwa team believes is required for Alex. DSA responded that while it does have nursing in one property, the nurses are not able to make decisions about the medications and vary the timing or dosages. She agreed that if Alex had funding for Nursing in his NDIS Plan, they could either recruit a nurse or I could purchase the service from another provider.

DSA emphasised the need for them to have comprehensive information before they could explore options in detail. It was agreed that the reports for Alex's plan review meeting on 10 February 2020 would be very helpful for DSA. DSA also explained how difficult it was to line up vacancies and funding for both SIL and SDA – not unlike the ACT.

We would not have been making these searches interstate except that the situation was desperate. The allied health manager had also articulated a list of requirements for a house for Alex which were consistent with robust SDA, which meant that ACT could not provide.

New doctor, new medicine

At this point of desperation and distress with Alex's condition, while we had no hope, a significant change occurred the next day! With Dr K on leave for a month, a relieving psychiatrist Dr N, with intellectual disability experience, wanted to make medicine changes for Alex. He wanted to add aripiprazole which had been shown to be advantageous previously, but this time as a depot (meaning as a long lasting form) addressing Alex's compliance issues, and lithium for the manic symptoms. He also wanted to remove Alex's valproate arguing he did not think Alex was having petit mal episodes. He might have thought aripiprazole was indicated for the mania but he was not explicit on this.

I think it was a mistake to make three changes at once. We needed to know the effect of one change on its own, if there were changes in Alex. Indeed, Alex did improve and very quickly. He had never been prescribed lithium previously so this was new territory. Dr N said he had made these changes in consultation with Dr K.

I did not obtain a rationale from Dr N for thinking that Alex did not have petit mal seizures. I do not know whether he used historical data or as Alex presented in the doctor's short time at Dhulwa. I would have thought that while Dr N was observing Alex, he would have been taking some valproate even if he was sometimes non-compliant, and therefore there would have been some masking of any seizures. What did he think he was seeing? Dr K resumed the valproate when he returned from leave, in any case.

New year 2021 held the best news in a long time. I took a week's holiday interstate to see my married son and his family. I had a video call with Alex in the first week of January. I gave warning to those extended family members who might hear the conversation, thinking Alex might start yelling. To my delight, Alex was great. He made good social conversation. When he could see people in the background, he asked who they were and other sensible questions. He showed no sign of distress that I was away without him.

The processes underway in order to obtain the Model of Care from the behaviour specialist and other documentation from Dhulwa to take to NDIA asking for additional funding was now approached with optimism. I was not so pleased when I saw the draft from the behaviour specialist as it emphasised Alex at his worst. They had used the only collated data available from Dhulwa. This was from all his aggressive episodes of 2020 and did not include the improvements with the change in medication since December 2020. The argument was that we were trying to convince NDIA that Alex needed the additional and later extraordinary funding for SDA and 2:1 care and we needed to manage the risks associated with him at his worst. I had to accept the picture painted of Alex even though I knew another Alex, and regardless of the causes of the bad behaviour.

The Model of Care concluded that Alex needed to live on his own, except for carers, and perhaps live with other clients later. The home needed to have three zones: one for Alex's private space with his bedroom, shared spaces with particular features of open plan in the kitchen area and office space for carers which could also double as a bedroom for a carer overnight as needed. The dwelling should be single story with robust fittings. These requirements could be expected to make it harder for Housing ACT to supply housing for Alex, but I think the stories of Alex from 2020 put Housing completely offside.

Included in Dhulwa's documentation for NDIA was a letter from Dr K from 4 February 2021 recommending that Alex be considered for funding for intensive support for living in the community. Dr K stated:

> Mr Cameron's psychotic symptoms have been stable for a considerable period of time, and recently he has been compliant with his medication and managing to avoid engaging in further episodes of interpersonal violence. The

treating team are of the opinion that Mr Cameron would strongly benefit from returning to live in the community in order to continue to actively work on achieving his recovery goals in a less restrictive environment. As Mr Cameron has now been in institutions for several years, he will need significant support to transition into the community again.

This represented a very different way of assessing Alex! It was discouraging, however, that Dr K only mentioned schizophrenia, did not mention the mania or schizo-affective disorder and there was no correlation of Alex's better mental health state with the recent changes in medication. In the next doctor's report to the Tribunal, the further omission of reference to benefits of different medication since the previous Tribunal hearing was painfully indicative of him not wanting to acknowledge that a different doctor's ideas might have been good ones.

A meeting on 5 February at Dhulwa, called a Secure Mental Health Services Allied Health Team Meeting, was attended by Dhulwa clinical and allied health staff, the social worker (new) and an administration officer, ACOS, the support coordinator, behaviour specialist, Senior Public Advocate, ISRP and me. Two Housing representatives also attended but when invited to contribute, neither was able to provide an update. Dr K noted Alex's reduction in assaults but did not mention correlation with medicine changes. The behaviour specialist's draft report had been circulated. The recommendation would be for robust fittings in any housing with consideration of applying for SDA in the preparation of the Model of Care.

Shock from Housing ACT

Subsequently, there was a housing meeting on 17 February chaired by ISRP. The Director of Housing ACT attended and was able to give an update! She announced suddenly that they now could not provide a house for Alex but they would continue in the whole of government approach which they said all along should be the way to deal with this responsibility. What did that mean? The government was divided into directorates each taking a field of activity, their responsibilities under the aims of the whole of government. So the government's public housing belonged to Housing ACT. The Director gave no explanation for why they wanted to assign Alex's housing needs to other Directorates, perhaps taking health funding for example.

My response via email to the group was:
- Why did it take 2 years for Housing to subsequently determine that Alex was ineligible for a tenancy?
- Why did Housing fail to communicate for long periods: not responding to phone calls from Alex's support coordinator, not attending several multi-agency meetings about Alex?
- Why did Housing leave the guardian to suffer under the fantasy all the time that Housing was still looking, so that early 2020 she agreed to a less-than-ideal accommodation rental for a planned discharge mid-2020 on the argument that it would only be temporary before the public housing was offered?
- When selected Housing staff did attend a meeting (at Dhulwa) and communicate (e.g. about a specific organisation managing the lease) towards the end of

2020, why was there no mention of this subsequent thinking and decision?
- Why has there been no formal communication to Alex (thus his Guardian) that this is Housing's decision, rather relying ad hoc on presentation at the meeting of parties convened by others, at a point of utter despair to find housing for Alex?

The Director of Housing sent me a long justifying email on 18 February including the following:

> The additional information Housing ACT has received regarding Alex's needs and requirements does not demonstrate that Alex is capable of independent living with the capacity to undertake a housing tenancy. This would also include the concerns that I had spoken about in relation to Housing ACT's ability to engage and support Alex and in turn the potential concerns regarding staff safety.
>
> As I have reiterated on numerous occasions throughout the case conferences, it is Housing ACT's view that a whole of Government response is required to find an appropriate housing solution for Alex.
>
> In addition to these aspects, I would also like to highlight that Housing ACT does not have any stock which would be suitable for Alex. As you are aware, Alex has very specific dwelling requirements which will require a 'bespoke' build.

When Alex was sent a letter approving housing in November 2018 their notion of independent living did not feature. He was not independently living anywhere up to then and was not expected to reside anywhere without support. If you need support from paid carers or family and friends does that mean you are not independently living according to Housing? Does that mean that public housing is never given to anyone relying on the NDIS funded supports? Why was Housing still talking about bespoke housing managed by them if Alex was declared ineligible across the board? I could see no logic or consistency in what Housing was saying. Why did they think they had to personally 'engage' with Alex? Did they not understand guardians and disability support?

Alex's new NDIS Plan 24 February included plenty of funds for continuing the search for suitable housing but without a discharge date, NDIA could not commit to a package for the support workers in the community yet. There could be no discharge date without a place for Alex to go.

The behaviour specialist and the allied health manager were shocked at Housing's stance. Too many times, I met barriers and systems that did not function. I was getting short on patience and politeness. I set about writing my third complaint – to the Human Rights Commission claiming discrimination against Alex because of his disabilities.

Chapter 10 Even if discharged, only by exile
March 2021- January 2022

My third Complaint to the Human Rights Commission included the following statements:

> My son (39 years this year) has been kept in a health facility since November 2017 except for brief efforts at discharge which proved insufficiently planned for and were poorly executed. His requirements for health care were prolonged because of incompetence in the mental health facilities in the ACT in managing patients with intellectual disabilities and autism. He has suffered poor mental health care, unnecessary lengthy periods of decline with as many different medical opinions as doctors that saw him in a passing parade, and disgraceful deterioration to his physical and dental health. Despite his complex conditions with ID and autism associated with a rare gene mutation, he has suffered a regime of judgment and punishment for difficult and at times aggressive behaviour, promoted by being kept in an environment working contrary to his framework for understanding the world. He has been at Dhulwa since February 2019.

My son is judged to be now medically ready for discharge. However, he is rendered homeless by an assessment that he cannot return home to live with me, his guardian, and requires a home that Public Housing seems self-satisfied to say it cannot provide him.

Public Housing has behaved disgracefully towards my son: after accepting his eligibility for housing and agreeing for him to have a three-bedroom house in 2018, it now refuses to provide any house. Why the change of mind? In the interval, while we waited with assurances that it was still looking, I could have explored other options and it could have built a house from scratch! Housing has denied my son these opportunities. It looks suspiciously as if they want to deny him a home so that someone else pays and in an arrangement in which it can claim SDA funding from NDIA – on the basis of the behaviour specialist report recently finalised.

We are applying for SDA for my son but will not know the decision for another couple of months. If solely relying on SDA and the associated build or modification, the so prescribed appropriate housing will take another two years. It is a human right issue to keep an intellectually disabled man in a forensic mental health facility at all but now he faces another two years in an extremely restrictive environment which bewilders and torments him. His wellbeing can only decline.

Could there please be a resolution to this appalling situation for my son? Shame on the ACT Government for its neglect of my vulnerable son.

The Public Advocate recently suggested that the decommissioned Extended Care Unit behind Calvary Hospital could be converted to a temporary home for my son. If this is the only way to discharge my son in an expeditious manner then I ask that this be agreed to as soon as possible. Time will be required to set this up of course, not least because a newly recruited and trained team of support workers 24/7 is required.

In conjunction with this possible means of getting discharge soon, assistance is required for a potential SDA developer to purchase land for a more long-term solution. Blocks of land appear to be difficult in the ACT where my son would prefer to live. The ACT Government should be willing to sell a block to an SDA developer capable of building to my son's requirements.

Housing has already proven itself to be difficult, poor at communication, unreliable and untrustworthy and I have little confidence that the Housing department with its current attitudes and culture (and limited resourcing) could manage what is required for my son. However, registered private SDA developers able to acquire suitable land offer a reasonable avenue to pursue.

The complaints process involves telling them what you have done to try to resolve the problem so I wrote:

> I have kept in touch with all the relevant parties to advocate for my son. I have attended meetings, prepared documents and telephoned as required. I have given a good part of the last three and a half years to advocacy in the circumstances of my son's needs for treatment and

appropriate care and the right to have a home. I submitted a complaint last year to try to improve the treatment and environment at Dhulwa in the tragic circumstances of his failure to be discharged then. I submitted to the Inquiry into abuse and neglect of people with a disability in the health system on the neglect by omission by the ACT Government to have the appropriate facilities and skills to care for those with a dual disability of intellectual disability and mental illness. I wrote to the Chief Psychiatrist trying to get reform. I wrote to two successive Ministers for Mental Health: Shane Rattenbury and then Emma Davidson and neither have replied, not even with an acknowledgement.

I have implored and begged and tried to make everyone aware of the torture my son experiences. There is still no resolution. My patience is wearing thin.

It would take months for the processes to ensue in response to this complaint and in the meantime, I could not stop trying every avenue for Alex, taking lack of help from Housing ACT as a given.

Valproate follow-up

Despite the dramatic improvement with Alex being given aripiprazole and lithium, by late January Dr K resumed and even increased valproate, coincident with some bad behaviour again. I was uncertain what was causing what. I had not forgotten my concerns with the use of valproate in Alex's medicine regime. I heard of a neuropsychiatrist visiting Canberra from Melbourne. She agreed to visit Alex and write a report. Permission was granted at Dhulwa for her review on 12 February.

The neuropsychiatrist thought that an adverse reaction of valproate would be possible but unlikely, and Alex's valproate levels did not seem to correlate with his outbursts. Valproate does have negative effects through the potential to increase ammonia in the blood which therefore this expert recommended Alex be monitored. I do not think it ever was. The neuropsychiatrist suggested catatonia (due to possibly a sudden drop in dopamine due to his mental illness) as a cause behind Alex's variability in behaviour. This report of April 2021 was provided to Dhulwa. I received no comment from Dr K or Dr L. No discussion on catatonia.

Recovery could not lessen the need for an SDA home

Alex had become overtly mentally unwell under ACT healthcare, leading to a record highlighting aggression and assaults, to be held up as the Alex to be catered for in the community. Discovery of how medication could be adjusted to get much of the old Alex back could not alter that record. Alex's die was cast. He had to move out of the ACT if he were to ever find community housing. He now had to carry the fixed burden of what healthcare had done to him either because of reputation, or in what his body was now doing. He carried the label they stuck on him. The ACT community had no facility to cater for this burdened Alex.

We could not think of giving up. Dr K had cycled back to saying Alex could be discharged. We were following two lines of securing accommodation for Alex during 2021: SDA and a temporary facility behind Calvary hospital, if it could be satisfactorily modified and rented from Canberra Health Services. We did not want to, and Alex did not want to have to, move interstate. If we were to get approval for SDA it was far preferable to be within ACT. Public Housing had only begun to think about SDA and as described, did not want Alex as a tenant anyway, every enquiry and effort to find an SDA developer within ACT failed and we made renewed efforts interstate. Whatever SDA we targeted, Alex would need temporary accommodation for about two years because it was unthinkable to leave him in Dhulwa for the time it took for an SDA to be built. We foolishly placed great store in the idea dangled in front of us to use the Health Service's old facility Extended Care Unit Villa D behind Calvary Hospital.

We had to engage a specialist writer in preparing an application to NDIA for SDA. We chose in February 2021 an organisation highly recommended as the best in the country. They would engage their own occupational therapist for an assessment to support the application. Hence, we started another round of discussions, ensuring that we passed on all the documents about Alex as previously written, and checking draft documents produced. The process took until July 2021, which required extra correction steps as each of the OT and the final report writers skewed some things from the existing reports. It took extra time in these steps because they insisted on sending only PDF versions which were harder to use for returning edits and corrections. NDIA undertook their approval in minimum time thankfully. We next had to find a vacancy in an SDA development, ideally one completed or well on the way.

The Director at Housing and their Branch Manager confirmed on 1 March their earlier decision and gave additional information about how they would take SDA money should Alex be approved by NDIA for SDA and something was built on a block of land Housing provided. A big issue at this meeting was understanding the implications of the SDA route no matter who was building: implications for Alex to be held at Dhulwa for another two years! On the negative side, Housing ACT would not consider giving a block of land unless its officers were satisfied that the tenancy and support worker risks were managed. Why did Housing think it could assess that separately from the professionals' risk assessments? Housing, in reality, gave conditions about tenancy management which would be no different for someone of Alex's disabilities taking any Housing tenancy. Was Alex treated differently for some reason?

Housing ACT was defensive in a letter to Karen Toohey, Discrimination, Health Services, Disability and Community Services Commissioner in May. I could see various things had been misinterpreted by Housing from their view of the world. Housing seemed to take the view that they were responsible for support worker safety in any public tenant's house. Essentially, Housing ACT stated it was the behaviour specialist's report that highlighted the gap between Alex's housing needs and Housing ACT's capacity to meet these needs.

Towards the end of the year when I still had no resolution to my complaint, I investigated taking the Directorates to court for violation of human rights. However, I wanted to only do things which would have a chance of getting Alex out of Dhulwa. I found out in October that an ACAT process would take too long and the alternative of going to the Supreme Court could be too costly for Alex and me. Lawyers I spoke to said there was a good case but I put my energies elsewhere.

My first grandchild was born in May 2021 for which I made a quick trip interstate. I told Alex about the birth cautiously as it was yet another family event in which he could not participate. He was interested but did not express anxiety about not being able to see his nephew.

Offer of disused accommodation went nowhere

The Villa D accommodation behind Calvary Hospital distraction occurred as follows:

At a meeting on 18 March 2021 between the Senior Public Advocate, the allied health manager and Dr K and me at Dhulwa, the Senior Public Advocate presented the idea of using the decommissioned building behind Calvary for a short-term solution. It was due for demolition in about two years but could be put to use in the meantime. Reception of this idea at Dhulwa was favourable and it was sent up the line in Canberra Health Services.

ISRP had stepped back but had participated in recent meetings. This has included leading two meetings with ACT Housing and Dhulwa to further explore the barriers, which were preventing Alex being provided with Housing in the ACT. Canberra Health Services proposed that the Office for Disability co-chair a cross government executive level group with them to solve his housing crisis, as this issue was said to sit more appropriately in the Office of Disability remit of service provision. Thus, there was supposed to be a mechanism for high level negotiations about accommodating Alex including the use of Villa D.

I had requested that approval for Alex's use of the decommissioned facility Villa D be determined as soon as possible. The 2021 timeline went something like this:

March: Idea mooted and sent up the line.

April: In principle OK, acknowledgement by Canberra Health Services that this was a good idea.

May: Visits and assessment by the behaviour specialist and the support worker organisation. Team produced a list of modifications required, categorised as essential or recommended. The allied health manager is made coordinator of the project. ISRP commits to helping with financial support if ball park figures could be given.

June: Health infrastructure responds with an excessive $100,000 required. Communication starts to fade. Questions about what this amount covers went unanswered. There was some talk about the most expensive item being the sewerage system because it was recommended in our list that certain bathrooms with their toilets be closed off. Infrastructure said you cannot just stop using toilets. The logic was obscure as of course no matter how many of the existing toilets Alex's stay would use, none were being used currently in the empty building. Quotes would be obtained for the modifications.

The estimate for modifications was large but was only a small proportion of what it was costing them to keep Alex at Dhulwa.

July: We kept waiting for answers. We offered to curb the list of modifications.

Six months after the idea was first aired, we were told by project coordinator (allied health manager#1) that all was progressing: Canberra Health Services would undertake a single select quoting process. It should not take very long. This was Immediately countered by the then Acting Executive Director emailing me that the single select process was for an architect to prepare a scope of works (on top of what we had already done on required modifications four months earlier). The project coordinator had been superseded. Further, the project coordinator was told she would no longer be part of the project.

So, the Acting Executive Director of Mental Health, Justice Health, Alcohol and Drug Services created an intervening step and potentially prolonged stages when we were seeking speedy resolution on a human rights issue. I did not forget how I was lectured on Alex's human rights when I declined an accommodation offer in January 2018 (I had a strong rationale). The Acting Executive Director sounded satisfied, representing this intervention as action forward, and as benevolence from Health committed money for the architect to expedite the project, but there was no talk of money for anything else at this stage.

If an architect step was really the most appropriate way forward in planning to spend public money, why did it take three months to come to this? There was never any project management from the start. There were unanswered questions about the anticipated process once the architect completed their work. For example, will the architect estimate the modifications costs or is that another step? How long before the request for quote(s) to do the modifications start?

I could see we were far from getting the quotes for the actual work and thus there would be no talks about ISRP involvement yet. We were in danger of retaining the Catch 22 in which Health will not be able to seek quotes if they do not know where the money will come from and ISRP will not be able to offer money if they do not know how much it will cost. Good people had tried to move this forward. Senior management badly let Alex down.

That is, we experienced another five months of Alex living in his idea of hell. And worse, it could take another five months even if 'progress' continues to be made. I was frustrated and disgusted.

The Acting Executive Director did not send me any updates after August and the person now acting as allied health manager #2 at Dhulwa did not seem to ever know much about it. There was no information from September to November. Third hand I heard that there was some sort of meeting of parties in October but no Scope of Works had been produced. At one stage there was mention of the wrong form being sent to Infrastructure and that a new submission on the correct form needed to be made. At a December meeting at Dhulwa the allied health manager #2 said there were no updates. After the meeting I heard that steps for the process had been identified and the completion date could be April 2022. By the time I heard there might have been movement to the next stage it was February 2022 and I just laughed.

I was livid when for the next doctor's report (February 2022) to the Tribunal, the author claimed that Health Services had been trying to find supported accommodation in Canberra including Villa D. There had been some investigations interstate by the Dhulwa social worker and follow up by the allied health manager in 2020 which was good but nothing compared to what Alex's support coordinator had done. More to the point, to claim good credentials for what was happening with Villa D was appalling. Whether this was a case of the author being told lies or it was deliberate spin to try to put Canberra Health Services in a good light, I thought this was really poor. Truth was needed for rational analysis to be able to find a way forward for Alex.

Frustration with the delay

Meanwhile, what was happening with our effort for housing through SDA? We turned into a blind alley time and again in this maze. We had tried ACT companies interested in SDA developments. Approval for robust standard dwellings had not been achieved with the existing projects. One ACT organisation that was thinking about building to robust standards answered my first call but the promised further calls never eventuated. A Queensland company seeking to expand to Canberra tried to work out a financially viable way to enter Canberra SDA. Unfortunately, the limited available land and zoning regulations made it financially impossible. We even tried to establish liaison between the Queensland company and the ACT relevant planning area but it all came to nothing.

I emailed the team on 9 August after finally visiting Alex when allowed with getting lockdown exemptions.

> It would break your heart to see his appearance: dishevelled hair to his shoulders, a hunched forward plod, nails either long or broken at the quick, and dirty clothes

and unshaven as lesser problems. At least it was only a day since his last shower. He said he was feeling unwell and tired. He was better cared for in his first year at Dhulwa when he was often aggressive. At least they let me come in with nail clippers and do his nails in the visiting room then.

After our work on medicine taking, I think we need work on personal hygiene that used to be so much better pre-hospital!

Departing went OK when the art therapist came – because she gently held his hand while I withdrew. Thankfully this was before the guards arrived. He was so tired during the visit that he was falling asleep mid-sentence. He kept shifting closer to me on the seat so he could rest on me as a pillow. I do not think he would get to art as he needed to sleep. He sobbed about getting out.

Five days later Alex's 39th birthday and his fourth while incarcerated was very quiet. He had expressed ideas about lots of people visiting, only to be very disappointed when this could not happen. He did, not understand the COVID restrictions. I kept seeing a very sleepy Alex. He was being over-medicated! Had they just forgotten him while he was not providing the same trouble?

Success in getting dental treatment

Concurrently, I was still concerned about Alex's teeth. After all the missed dental appointments the previous year, we were able to make progress from seeing Alex's private dentist in March to getting Alex to a specialist periodontist. I thought the specialist might say it would be too hard to help Alex because of the gradual loosening of many teeth and the situation Alex was in was not conducive to good dental care. Nonetheless, he decided he would do implants and crowns, but only under anaesthetic which meant trips to hospital for Alex.

The treatment required two hospital surgery visits, one in May and the other in August. It was a success but with a few problems on the way. I was given permission to be at both private hospital visits provided I was gone when Alex awoke so that he would not think I was taking him home. The first hospital day surgery created a few problems for the hospital where the procedure was undertaken in the absence of communication about what kind of patient Alex was. Fortunately, there was a sensible and kindly security guard on duty whom Alex adopted as a friend. The guard was able to calm Alex and see him through to the time of moving to the theatre. The nurse wanted him to take his clothes off not anticipating the fuss this would cause. We managed a compromise.

Once Alex was in theatre, he resisted the anaesthetist doing his work. Alex was given options. He rejected a mask and then had to be coaxed to cooperate with a venepuncture. The periodontist had a fantastic manner with Alex and won him over. Then Alex's veins would not cooperate and it took three tries. Amazingly, Alex was calm through all this but it delayed the theatre work. They had no time left to put in the temporary crowns hoping to make use of the anaesthetic for this too. They said that Alex could come to the dentist's rooms for these later but this was thwarted. Alex was not able to attend the dentist rooms appointment for temporary crowns because of staff shortages at Dhulwa on the appointment day. He had to pay for the crowns nonetheless because they had been made by the specialist.

The second session to theatre for the permanent crowns in August went better after the earlier lessons were learnt.

Search interstate inevitable

In September 2021 the Behaviour Specialist wrote an addendum to account for Alex's improvements. This was too late for Housing ACT and too late for avoiding the need to move Alex out of ACT. Exile was inevitable.

I investigated several SDA developments or planned developments in Victoria. These developments usually occur where new land is made available. Sometimes an SDA build can occur after demolition of an older dwelling. I investigated Koo Wee Rup in Eastern Victoria which was only on the planning board. I applied for a place for Alex in a development in Small Town, Western Victoria where the developers had started to build three units on a double block near the centre of the town. We were lucky that there was one vacancy remaining and despite the waiting list, Alex was successful in September 2021. Plans were already approved so the time before completion should be much shorter. Success!

At last, with Alex's mental illness treated, discharge looked like it was really possible. Something was finally working for Alex. I put a lot of time into securing a Victorian based Support Coordinator and a Victorian Support Worker organisation. We planned how we could tell Alex and handle his disappointment that he would move away from ACT. We sent Alex pictures of the town and region and of new stages in building the units. Then the delays were communicated. COVID-19 had interrupted many constructions at the time. At least this company had already been able to store materials so was not going to suffer materials shortage. To our dismay, the completion date was put back many times.

Thus, Alex's discharge was put back and back. The team asked if he could get temporary or respite ACT accommodation in the interim. I had planned to move to Victoria too. I did not want Alex to feel I was abandoning him. I sped up my consideration of how I would do that and decided to rent a place which could help Alex move sooner while we waited for the SDA to be completed. Alex was so much better so this should work in the community now. I was excited to find a nice house in Small Town itself and took out a twelve month lease from Christmas 2021. It had plenty of bedrooms for disability staff and for me to visit while I swapped between ACT and Victoria for all the arrangements. I arranged for my guardianship order to be recognised in Victoria.

In October Alex was taken again to Canberra Hospital with cellulitis again. Again, he was placed on antibiotics and returned to Dhulwa. Alex was also given antifungal medication because of the state of his feet. This should not have been given orally because of an interaction with clozapine. Once this was realised, he was only given topical antifungals.

Alex kept complaining strongly from about November of being chilled by the air coming through the hospital air conditioning units. He had not complained of this the previous summer. He kept putting on more and more layers of clothes and while sweating even more profusely, would say he was freezing. We tried periods of stopping the fans to the air outlets but that was not sustained. It was a constant battle for the nurses. There was no cause of this shift mooted. I suppose in many ways it seemed just an extension of Alex's usual need to wear lots of layers for either warmth over winter or proprioception (comfort through cocooning).

I went through all the medical care Alex would need in Victoria including a GP, leg and foot care, a dentist for his ongoing tooth loosening needs and an ophthalmologist for the cataract that had developed in his right eye. I made enquiries about specialists. On the all-important mental health, we uncovered which public clinic would be responsible in that area and I asked Alex's ACT community GP for a referral to a local private psychiatrist with intellectual disability qualifications to be able to give advice. We made enquiries with the Victorian Dual Disability unit for what might be possible in supporting the responsible Mental Health Unit with Alex's complexity.

I also wanted Alex to see a neurologist. Apart from the issue of valproate never entirely preventing petit mal seizure episodes, Alex had been fainting and collapsing according to hospital reports. Dhulwa doctors had concluded these were attention-seeking episodes. They thought Alex had learnt that he could get visits to Canberra Hospital for tests so was faking these episodes to try and get there. I very badly wanted alternative care for Alex!

Poor handover from Dhulwa to Victoria

The referral from Dhulwa to the Regional Health Service running the Victorian Mental Health Unit was problematic. From December and over Christmas I could not get any confirmation of what was happening. Then I heard that Dr K was told that this Mental Health Unit would not take Alex. I said they had to because Alex now had an address in Small

Town Victoria. I asked how they had come to this opinion. I demanded of the allied health manager #3 and Dr K during a January phone call whether they had told the Victorian Mental Health Unit that Alex was a monster?! I was assured that a quite normal straightforward referral had been sent. I responded that I would not know this because I had not been sent a copy. They then sent me a copy which indeed did not say much – when it should have given a more complete picture and a more comprehensive handover.

Dhulwa had told the relevant Victorian Regional Health Service in its referral letter that:

> Currently his mental state is relatively settled and, no psychotic symptoms have been noted since his clozapine treatment was stabilised. Historically he has been prone to episodes of significant aggression and violence, however these have been significantly reduced during the last few months. Whilst on occasion he does experience episodes of frustration and become verbally aggressive, his behaviour has only infrequently proceeded to physical aggression, and he is able to de-escalate with assistance from staff.

Problems with these words are obvious to me: there was no mention of manic symptoms linked to no acknowledgement that clozapine was not enough, even if better than other antipsychotics such as olanzapine for the psychotic markers; and a big problem with the low precision and misleading term "historically" – this perhaps implies persistent, since childhood, or perhaps it means on one occasion but a long time ago or perhaps it has expanded implications as would "it is common knowledge". It was no wonder that the Victorian Regional Health Service blamed intellectual disability.

I wondered what the conferring doctors had said verbally. Dhulwa really preferred to be able to send Alex to another secure facility in Victoria but was told that a referral would have to come from the relevant Victorian local mental health unit, not Dhulwa. Dr K had no faith that Alex's placement in Small Town was a good idea. Dr K might have said discouraging things to the Mental Health Unit about Alex's needs, hoping it would refuse to be responsible for him. This was important to reflect on later in 2022. The subsequent quick assessment by the Victorian Mental Health Unit that Alex was only having settling and aggression problems once in Victoria because he was autistic, did not seem to come from their own independent assessment.

Alex's community team made direct approaches to the Victorian Mental Health Unit and found that it had not been given any information on the plans for Alex in the community. Dhulwa did not give any idea of the extensive support arrangements to be executed, including for blood tests and administration of all medication. This was not what we regarded as an appropriate handover of a complex patient.

Alex's behaviour specialist found that the Victorian Regional Health Service had not been given key documents in the referral process from Dhulwa such as the Model of Care and Transition Plan. They had not been given the opportunity, while they came to their intention to reject him, to consider the supports that Alex would have in place. Dhulwa had given them the impression that the clozapine clinic would have to supervise Alex's medicine taking daily, for which of course they did not have the resources. Arrangements for disability support workers to undertake this responsibility are normal and were in train for Alex.

I started the process of setting up the rental house travelling back and forth between ACT and Small Town. I arranged for white goods and a few furniture items so I could stay there. There would be enough space in the rental for much of Alex's things ready for the move to the SDA so I planned a removalist's van for January 2022.

Plans thwarted

Then disaster! All the previous troubles and torments were suddenly insignificant. Alex's life was in danger. Canberra Hospital rang me to tell me he was taken to the Emergency Department and then to ICU. I was back in Canberra and with COVID exemptions to visit him, sped to the hospital on 11 January 2022.

Alex was diagnosed with Neuroleptic Malignant Syndrome (NMS) which meant his body was burning up with potential organ shutdown, due to a relatively rare reaction to his antipsychotic medication. When he first went to Emergency it was thought he had pneumonia, which might have been true as I found out later it can be associated with NMS. Because I mentioned Alex's scary story with ketamine, they used droperidol to calm him. He was treated with antibiotics. The ICU doctor later told me he had stopped Alex's antipsychotics and lithium and that the Emergency droperidol was contraindicated for someone with NMS!

All I could think of was that, if he survived, Alex would be unable to be treated at all and would thus be forever psychotic and shut away for the rest of his life. I told the ICU doctor he needed to be aware of what Alex was now committed to: a shocking life. At best I thought we might have to repeat the horrible journey of the last few years from the start. Could Alex bear such torture? I was weighed down with trying to find his voice to act as his guardian.

No one from Dhulwa rang me to talk about what chances there were of getting Alex back on antipsychotics and the possible pace of such action. That might have been too kind. I had to suffer the agony. Even when the Canberra Hospital psychiatrist rang me, he left out this sort of important information. And that was even after he listened to me wailing about this as a total catastrophe.

Alex was blissfully unaware of anything except his physical problems. His high temperature, his increasing incontinence as a reaction to the loss of antipsychotics and his pressure sores over a large area of his buttocks. I nursed him every day for his stay in ICU and in the medical ward. The hospital seemed glad of my help in ICU with COVID-induced nursing shortages. He was then sent to a medical ward. At that stage, a rebound psychosis had not set in; instead he was very sociable and cooperative in the lull before the storm.

They managed to get him back to Dhulwa prior to a full-blown psychosis, but not before he had a bad day being brought back to the ward after escaping through the front door. This was a reaction to my departure for the afternoon because I had a meeting. I had been less careful about my words on saying goodbye because Alex had been so easy until then. Apparently, Alex thought I was saying I was not wanting to be his Mum when I said he should not be repeatedly calling "Mum" as I got to the door when I needed to leave. This was possibly the earlier stages of a rebound.

Alex had to return to Dhulwa with his catheter still in place to return later to attempt removal. After a failed trial-of-void with removal, he was kept one day to the side of ED while they waited for a specialist to reinsert a catheter. I stayed with him. He was manic and loud but not impossible. Late at night they brought him forward to a bed for the procedure, there were bunches of nurses standing ogling him, giggling. I thought even if these are not mental health nurses, this was not professional. Do they have to be explicitly told this is someone who is ill, mental ill yes but ill, and should not be disrespected?

The reinsertion meant that he had to be returned to Canberra Hospital urology clinic as an outpatient at a suitable time. I came to possibly assist. No one had planned for a psychotic patient to come to the clinic, the nurse could not handle it, and Alex was taken to the psychiatric intake assessment area as part of ED. He was agitated and not listening to me. Alex had been accompanied by a new Deputy Director of Nursing who had recently started. So key people at Dhulwa did not know Alex at this stage: the allied health manager and the Deputy Director of Nursing. The Clinical Nurse Consultant was still acting in the position after multiple changes over the years. Fortunately, Dr M who knew Alex well from Dhulwa was able to come to lead the situation.

At first Alex was cooperative and social with some nurses. By the evening, he was a nightmare and caused a lot of damage. He did manage to void his bladder though, to everyone's relief. I had been brought to the area in case I could be used to influence Alex but was kept out of his sight. Dr M chose to keep me hidden as the incident escalated. It was traumatic to see Alex so ill.

The nurses at Dhulwa did not seem to be prepared for Alex with a full rebound psychosis. One nurse whom Alex had grown to like, and who had been his nurse from the beginning at Dhulwa, was no longer rostered to be with him. He tried to say hello or wave when he could see her through the glass panelling in another ward. She would not now even acknowledge him. He was bewildered and hurt. I suspect he was violent with her, alienating her I am sure, but he had no understanding, once he was being re-medicated, of what had happened.

Alex was able to be started on clozapine again fairly quickly but a work up had to be used, of course. I was more hopeful. He was not resumed on aripiprazole which was stopped at the end of 2021 without anyone telling me. The argument now was that with the risk of NMS, "polypharmacy" was unwise. Lithium had been dropped as a potentiator of NMS and was now regarded as unusable for Alex ever. Dr K let the administration of aripiprazole lapse in November before there was any suggestion of NMS so I knew he was always against using it. Whenever I mentioned it, I was told by the current allied health manager that clozapine was the "main one" so that is all Alex needed. I regarded this as a non-clinical statement which showed no appreciation of possible qualitative differences between antipsychotic types. Dhulwa seemed to think that psychosis treatment was a matter of just filling up the tank, not being able to approach different neurotransmitters with nuance.

I also thought that not all patients should be regarded as the same. Dr K had commented to me once in 2021 that he did not prescribe with his patients the new medications that Alex had been put on. This was a worrying statement indicating he thought all Dhulwa patients were expected to be the same.

Could we salvage a discharge?

I was worried about discharge planning even with the resumption of clozapine. Dhulwa was only in favour of Alex going to another secure facility if moving to Victoria. Dhulwa seemed to like their control of discharge (through the PTO) to keep patients away from the community while they went through the motions of treating him, as if time in a restrictive environment did not matter. Dr K's narrative was focussed on Alex's tendencies to aggression and violence since the removal of his antipsychotics, not his potential to be better as he had been during 2021. Finally, Dr K had never absorbed any advice about Alex's manic symptoms but rather was party to blaming his intellectual disabilities and autism, which were untreatable pharmaceutically, while at the same time seeing only nurses as capable of caring for Alex safely.

Dr K did not engage in discussions with me about diagnoses and treatment, leaving me to work my own way through the theories. In the absence of being given explanations, I could only try to use what information I had and my own thinking to rationalise what was happening with Alex. I only found out recently that clozapine could have contributed to his repetitive and OCD-like behaviours. It would have been appropriate to discuss this with me in relation to pre- and post-commencement of clozapine, particularly when so many different doctors kept wanting to treat, unsuccessfully and potentially harmfully, his OCD.

After three years in Dhulwa it seemed to me that Dr L and Dr K would have a theory about why Alex was not getting back to his early 2017 state, living in the community with no, or manageable, problems and participating in many activities. Towards the end of one meeting in which Dr K was present I said no one from Dhulwa had convinced me that Alex was suffering from a neurodegenerative condition. "No" was Dr K's response. There was no more discussion. This could have meant that we would consider that or they had considered it already and, either did not come up with the evidence or found evidence to the contrary. It could have meant it was beyond their expertise.

Dr K was also not a team player, either with other health professionals or with the cross-disciplinary discharge team. On more than one occasion after a discharge team meeting about what and how to frame messages to Alex, Dr K would reveal something to Alex contrary to our decisions. Unprepared, I would be faced with Alex telling me that he was told something by Dr K for my response in keeping with what the team had decided.

Alex frequently reported to me over the next year how Dr K told him all these things were happening to him because he hurt me by throwing burning oil at me. Whether Dr K used those words or not, that was what Alex heard. It was untrue in both the nature of my injury and the reason for him being in mental health facilities. Alex would go on to tell me he loved me and would not hurt me. He tried to make sense of his predicament. "It was not supposed to be this way Mum!" he would exclaim in desperation as he sought to live the life he had always envisioned. I reflected that ACT mental health treatment had not managed to take away his spirit for wanting a life of family, friends, work and hobbies – so far. For example, Alex persisted with his dream to set up his own business mowing lawns. He said it would be called *Grassbusters* and he designed his advertisements to be put in letterboxes as flyers. He kept telling me of his worry that too many people were getting artificial lawns!

Chapter 11 Out of the frying pan.....

February 2022 - September 2022

The next ACT Tribunal Hearing was approaching in February 2022. I engaged a solicitor for Alex to help with an anticipated fight with Dhulwa at that Hearing. The Public Advocate and I made separate submissions while the solicitor prepared the legal arguments. The Public Advocate wanted to be clear that Alex needed to be in the least restrictive environment even with the need to be maintained on antipsychotic medication. He had been in Dhulwa far too long and they had reached a point of saying he was ready for discharge before he had contracted NMS. The Public Advocate wanted clear planning and their continued involvement for independent oversight.

I argued:

- The Dhulwa doctor's report for the Tribunal is biased and misleading.
- Dhulwa has a culture of avoiding planning for health and discharge of patients: more accountability for rehabilitation is required.
- Alex is sensitive to environment which in itself is a trigger for irritability and bad behaviour,

- He suffers from prolonged social isolation and will never get well while kept in Dhulwa.
- The idea of indefinite incarceration is intolerable for Alex, his mother and family.

His solicitor submitted that there was significant evidence which supported the best available treatment for Alex and treatment that would promote his recovery would be provided in the community. In addition, she submitted that there was significant evidence which identifies that the arrangement of Alex residing in Dhulwa was not the best available treatment, care or support for Alex and his individual needs. Indeed, the approach to care of Alex at that time was detrimental to his recovery.

She echoed the sentiments of the Public Advocate's concerns regarding the Dhulwa report and its apparent focus on Alex only since his ill health in January 2022 which resulted in him being taken off his antipsychotic medication. There was evidence as demonstrated by the consulting Behaviour Specialist that generally prior to January 2022, there was a "significant reduction in Alex's presentation of behaviours of concern". Was he not supposed to be returned to that state of health? If not, why not?

She acknowledged that there were ongoing discussions with the Victorian Regional Health Service as to the care of Alex. Despite such discussions, there would be an obligation for such health services to take over the care for Alex. The doctor's report was short on what the risks in the community actually were, so there was no evidence before the Tribunal that any Order should prevent Alex relocating

The solicitor had spoken to Alex and reported that he was miserable in Dhulwa. He indicated that he did not have enough to do and he wanted to go for a walk. He was distressed about the confines of his current position and indicated that if he were able to reside in the community, he would want to make friends and play basketball.

The solicitor asked for a two months' PTO only, instead of the usual six months, which would allow time for review after Alex's clozapine had been stabilised and time for recruitment and training of the prospective support workers in Victoria.

The Tribunal granted a four months' Order. The Tribunal noted that all involved in Alex's care would work expeditiously and jointly to negotiate an appropriate transfer to Victorian Mental Health facilities once the clinical situation allows. If any party sought a transfer order, this could be heard on the next occasion, and regard would be had for the factors under section 289 of the Mental Health Act 2015.

Dhulwa only interested in removing Alex from its care

It seemed to me that the feelings expressed through this Tribunal process caused Dhulwa to wash their hands of anything further on Alex's health. Staff kept saying from then on that nothing was going to prevent his discharge, not even some further assault incidents which seemed to highlight his lack of readiness for discharge. Not even the fuss they created about me visiting him at Dhulwa. If I was regarded as unsafe with him, how did they assess his safety in the community? Were they interested in assessing him and making medicine adjustments accordingly? It seemed that Dhulwa just wanted

Alex gone and I naively thought he could get better treatment anywhere but at Dhulwa.

New senior staff did not know Alex and were learning from scratch. They were only seeing Alex in his new phase post NMS and only being treated with clozapine and valproate. They would not have known Alex when well. As explained earlier, I had never been privy to any discussion from Dhulwa correlating certain treatments with Alex's mental state and behaviour so it could be that these staff had no insight on this either. The Deputy Director of Nursing was also new to Dhulwa rules and, keen to see some changes, invited me to see Alex in the ward (no other patients) rather than the visitors' room. This worked well on one occasion but not the next.

I had a very distressing visit to Dhulwa before they banned me altogether. Alex got anxious when it came time for me to leave. His mood was escalated over his MP3 player not working. I made the mistake of picking it up when I thought he was distracted. He snatched it from me and wanted to fix it himself. To prevent me from leaving he put his arm around my neck. This was uncomfortable but not threatening harm. The nurses wanted to separate us and rush me to the door. A different nurse came in with intent. They tried their trick of pretending to mess with his things in his room. I was horrified and would not budge. I said that is just trickery. I asked for time to let Alex calm down. They could not wait long enough. They made another move to distract Alex and then the new nurse pushed me to the door. I was furious at being manhandled. I protested loudly to the Clinical Nurse Consultant who was seeing me out, explaining the history behind my objections to the trickery and how I would rather have Alex's arm around my neck than be pushed by a nurse. They did not appear to have my wellbeing in mind.

Dhulwa was concerned, however, about their Duty of Care which was so often thrown at me. What they were referring to was duty to the public and effecting a discharge so that any risk Alex posed could be disassociated with them or ACT Health. They planned and considered, re-planned and re-thought. Eventually the decision was to fly Alex to a Victorian regional airport with nurses and security guards. Never mind the expense, he would be out of their jurisdiction and bypass New South Wales altogether. Alarm bells should have been ringing that this extreme process was not for someone well enough after the NMS episode for community living under the care of a mental health unit not properly briefed.

For the June Tribunal Hearing the doctor's report included the following:

> There is significant risk of harm to other people including property damage and physical and verbal aggression/violence. Although the frequency of aggressive/violent behaviour has reduced, he is ongoing risk of aggressive behaviour towards other people. Despite his recent improvement he continues to display episodes of aggression, such as charging toward staff on the 4/6/2022 and following a maintenance worker and preventing access to his room 7/6/2022.
>
> He has previously been observed to engaged in self harm including punching or slapping his head.
>
> He is dependent on staff for his activities of daily living, and to manage his complex medical comorbidities such as

chronic cellulitis. There is significant risk of deterioration of his physical health without appropriate support from staff.

We seek a two month order to cover the period of time until Mr Cameron can be transferred interstate, and to allow for the possibility that unforeseen events could delay his transfer. Once his discharge date is known with certainty, we intend to request that his treatment order be revoked.

So, the significant risk of harm to others etc. was not enough to prevent discharge but any occurrence of unforeseen events could. I was frustrated with this logic. I wanted Alex out of Dhulwa. Events would prove that his move to Victoria was fatal, but I do not think he would have improved in Dhulwa. He was not going to improve while his mental illness symptoms were not recognised.

I submitted to the June Tribunal that the relevant Regional Health Service in Victoria had agreed to take Alex (email from them attached to my submission) and that Victoria would not need a Treatment Order (as per a second email attached). The Tribunal agreed that as soon as Alex was transferred their order would be revoked.

There were further delays with the SDA build. If Alex were to be discharged in July, he had the option of using the private rental, provided I could make it work. A few modifications were required to make it more robust for him and quickly. I was in Small Town for this and engaged tradesmen to carry out works such as installation of safety glass film on the lower windows. I also had the glass shower door in the main bathroom removed and kept in the garage for re-installation later. The agent inspected the property late June. She did not comment about the bathroom hand-rails I had installed, on backboards for strength, but did ask me about the shower door. I explained that my son was coming and since he was a big man with disabilities, I thought it safer. The agent was satisfied and commented that the house was being well maintained. It was to be November 2022 before the SDA was completed.

The big move

The date of 4 July was agreed for the transfer. We had a plan for who should accompany him and who should meet him at the airport. I was to be at the Small Town house while staff from the support worker organisation drove him from the airport. The driver of the van for this was Alice a Support Worker Coordinator who had met Alex in Canberra and had several video calls with him so he should have felt comfortable with her.

There was an incident at the airport. Alex wanted to take pictures with his camera. Security wanted him off the area. Alex's pants fell down with nothing to hold them up once he took his hand to the camera. The situation escalated. Alice had to fight to get Alex into the van. She took off feeling like she was in command of a getaway car. We do not know who was briefed or not briefed but it could have got very ugly.

Alex would not get out of the van at Small Town at first. When he did, he crouched in the foetal position on the nature strip. I crouched down with him for ages while neighbours peered and looked worried. Alex had been petrified.

The settling in did not go well. It was only when Alex got to the house that we realised how unwell he really was. I will give a detailed log of events, some with associated status reports I crafted at the time, for the next two months' struggle. This detail is needed for the reader to understand how we were out of the frying pan into the fire for Alex's escape from Dhulwa. I could hear Dr K all the way from Canberra saying, "I told you the Regional Health Service did not want to look after Alex."

I visited the house often but did not want to overshadow the need for care workers to be able to develop relationships with Alex. It was difficult in circumstances for which we did not want him to feel abandoned in exile. Sometimes I would be there in the afternoon or evening when Alex wanted to lie down. I would sit by the bed. He would say, even though exhausted, "I do not want to go to sleep because when I wake up you will be gone".

The Support Coordinator (and meeting organiser), the Behaviour Specialist, the Support Worker Organisation, the relevant mental health unit and I comprised the Care Team for Alex. We met weekly but the mental health unit could not always attend.

The start of trouble

9 July – Alex ran in front of several moving cars on a nearby busy road and refused to stop. I was with him and found him unresponsive to my requests not to keep charging at cars. Alex was taken to the nearest Regional Hospital Emergency Department via ambulance. In this hospital the Mental Health Triage team advised that Alex should have been taken to the

smaller hospital close to Alex's Mental Health Unit an hour's drive away. The Regional Hospital said that "Alex will never be admitted to our hospital or the Mental Health Centre for Psychiatric Help." This was contrary to the agreed Crisis Management Plan for Alex and reflected a denial that Alex needed psychiatric help.

I recognised an ongoing problem with reliance on new people all the time who did not know the 'well' Alex. I wrote to the whole team including our clinical contact at the Mental Health Unit. I explained:

> Alex of today is not the best Alex can be. I know a very different Alex not exhibiting these symptoms. I do not believe his medication is the best it could be knowing that he has had better results previously, prior to the commencement of his admissions from November 2017.
>
> Alex will not be able to live in the community whilst he keeps thinking people are calling him names. He is only going to get angry and then heightened and aggressive.
>
> Could we have a review earlier than I thought I would ask for one. I had not realised how manic he is. His psychotic symptoms are not under control despite his clozapine.
>
> The first thought might be that he is just missing the valproate this week. I do not believe now, however, that even when he was compliant with taking the valproate whilst at Dhulwa that he was right with respect to psychotic symptoms post January. Another idea might be that he is finding everything very strange in a new place.

Signs of mania

Please note these excursions of Alex into lots of chuckling while telling the stories such of the movie "Home Alone" etc. are not the Alex of old.

My list of symptoms of concern:

- hours of excited talk
- swapping quickly from one subject to another without a breath
- swapping to teary emotional talk quickly.
- Paranoia/delusions or just hearing voices: the persistence that the neighbours are calling him retard and spastic. Delusions about being a radio announcer, about being able to learn to drive a car etc. Perseveration on the hurts he has experienced at Dhulwa and not being able to live as we were in 2017.

Brief history of medicine changes since 2017

- Stable years from 2009 on clozapine, aripiprazole and valproate (low dose clozapine) Aripiprazole added by psychiatrist who thought Alex had unusual features that might benefit from the pharmacology of a partial agonist.
- Increased valproate mid 2017 because of petit-mal seizures (? the start of the hell)
- November 2017 admission - accidently left out aripiprazole despite being shown his Webster pack with it included.

- Readmission December persisted omission, doctors denying mistake and compounded poor care by removing clozapine.
- On surprise he became psychotic, resumed antipsychotics with olanzapine despite this being shown to be less than adequate over a decade previously. Manic symptoms not recognised because after all - he has ID and autism so of course he behaves "funny".
- No resumption of clozapine until 2020. No aripiprazole. Valproate dosing during this time I am unsure of.
- Christmas 2020 three changes: removal of valproate, addition of lithium and addition of aripiprazole as depot. Dramatic improvement resulted - could not tell to which change this could be attributed.
- February-March 2021 resumption of valproate.
- Sedation high through 2021 but I did not see him much because of COVID restrictions. Serious exhibition of something wrong with claims of feeling extremely cold Nov-Dec. Emergency admission in January and diagnosed with NMS.
- Removal of clozapine and lithium with subsequent resumption of clozapine only, Aripiprazole stopped but it seems to have occurred in late 2021. No information despites requests.

Increases in dosage of clozapine with worries not therapeutic levels, accounting for hearing voices. Is that the whole story of this year? I have not been kept up to date. It seems that even with higher doses Alex is hearing voices and the other symptoms as set out above. Dhulwa thought it was "better" with dosing him once per day in the mornings.

Fears of return of NMS. Fears he will never live in community. Who is in charge of determining the balance?

I had to write these thoughts down. It has been hard to have a voice on these matters through this transition period.

This email was ignored. I tried sending it to a psychiatric nurse at the clinic on 26 July having found out that the first contact was on leave and there was, perhaps, no forwarding of emails to stand-in staff. I did not receive an out of office email. It had been hard to have good communications with Dhulwa for months and now the Mental Health Unit was going to be even more difficult.

> *I Really Have Had a fucking very Bad time there, So all you Jack Sickoes are just are very Nasty there all Butt for all Only The Man Nurse [name deleted] the Right Good Nurse, there, So you all there are Pieces of dirt there, only, Because that Nurse There is only for my Eyes only, so suck Brick All you other Sicko Men There And All of you other Bad Mean, Nasty, Horrible and Very Bad Disgusting Violent other Lady, Men And Doctor and Nurses There, Because it was my very own very Nasty State of Shock Shit head Place to Be Because yous are Really Suck into Dipshit far Trouble Disgusting Stuff, Morons...*
>
> *...Now you all Listen to me i Very Much hated the fecking way yous all did Treat me like Dirt*

Alex stayed up at night writing whilst manic, mainly to express his hatred of Dhulwa. This text reveals his emotion and rush of words due to mania.

Alex was discharged on 750 mg clozapine daily when the doctor's notes to the Tribunal had said Dhulwa was aiming for a return to 500 mg daily with Alex's workup. No one had ever told me this increased dose would be used and certainly gave me no rationale. As his valproate dose was also raised, I suspected that the increase in clozapine was to cover the increased metabolism due to valproate.

Despite my and carer's requests no health help was provided

The following timeline for July to September indicates the lack of help from the Mental Health Unit which was fixated on Alex's disabilities, particularly autism, for some reason, but not on their supposed area of expertise: mental illness. Alice told them Alex's current bad behaviour was not due to autism (with which she had years of experience) and I sent a copy of an expert's letter to the Mental Health Unit, trying to put the inclusion of 'autism' in Alex's diagnosis in context. This log also represents the start of some nastiness from the townsfolk and the local police, who should have known better. The Mental Health Unit psychiatrist, Dr O, was holding off on urgent treatment required because Alex needed to settle!

11 July – Police correspondence re: multiple complaints from the community regarding Alex. Residents wish to take out intervention orders.

Review of Alex by Psychiatric Nurse from the mental Health Unit – advised no doctors available to conduct review and I noted – "he was at pains to say Alex's autism obscured the interpretation of his behaviour which was probably not due to mental illness."

18 July – Review with Mental Health Unit Psychiatric Nurse. No change in approach.

19 July – I emailed the contact Psychiatric Nurse at the Mental Health Unit and wrote:

> I reiterate my concerns using the following record of my conversation with Dr O, consultant Psychiatrist at the Mental Health Unit for Small Town.
>
> Dr O was adamant that more time was required for Alex to settle and for observations before he would change medication (antipsychotics and mood stabilisers?) but would re-consider the PRN.
>
> I stated my dissatisfaction that all Alex's current behaviours are being ascribed to autism. He agreed that was not the case. I referred to the letter from the Sydney dual disability psychiatrist in 2009 not even favouring the diagnosis of autism in 2009. He had not heard of Dr Sydney Expert so I presume you did not pass on my information.
>
> I stated more than once to Dr O that Alex's manic symptoms are not a stress response. He had exhibited manic symptoms whilst in hospital from the time his antipsychotics were withdrawn in late 2017 and in his period of instability in 2008 but not in the intervening years. He was showing many episodes of mania during 2018. Thus, it is not a continuous feature of his presentation but associated with inadequate medication.

Further he can exhibit much happy mania using giggling and notions of making movies without irritability and aggression. His manic symptoms did not just arise with the stress of the move to Victoria.

The ONLY period whilst hospitalised since 2017 in which Alex was showing good behaviour was during 2021 whilst on lithium and aripiprazole with clozapine. The poor state at discharge whilst only on clozapine, albeit with mostly taken valproate, was only evident to us after discharge and was not supposed to represent the best Alex could be. There again is evidence of reliance on clozapine alone being insufficient to remove all manic symptoms.

I made reference to two possible contributions to Alex's fluctuations of mood whilst compliant with clozapine administration, apart from excitements and anxieties about events: valproate, currently sometimes taken, can increase the metabolism of clozapine, and Alex is sporadically vomiting but at times not tracked to know how close to dose administration.

Dr O acknowledged that aripiprazole has the advantage of being retained sufficiently for a day of missed dosage to be acceptable.

In discussing the risk that Alex portrays if no further medication change is undertaken, Dr O expressed his view that Alex was currently OK to be managed by the Support Worker Organisation because so far, he has been kept out of hospital. [Emphasis added]

Dr O said he was thinking about changing PRN, probably increasing the dose of lorazepam. He asked me had Alex ever taken quetiapine at Dhulwa, which I answered in the affirmative, but it was unclear why it was stopped or what marker of success or otherwise Dhulwa was using anyway. Dr O did not say it was as PRN he was contemplating quetiapine.

Dr O said he was making the referral to Victorian Dual Disability Service next week.

I reiterate that closer monitoring of Alex's risk is required and not just by using the criterion of being kept out of hospital. This is particularly obvious after hearing the police's attitude.

27 July – I provided historical communication to the Mental Health Unit from Alex's dual disability psychiatrist from Sydney from 2018, playing down the role of autism in Alex's presentation.

29 July – Victorian Police called the Support Worker Organisation on-call number – recommended Alex be put in an institution and asked, 'if Alex declines medication, why can't he be injected?'

Late July: nothing from the Mental Health Unit.

The next Care Team Meeting 4 August (to which we invited the Mental Health Unit but no representative attended), discussed Alex's presentation: staff observing, "responding to internal stimuli, paranoia, mood rapidly fluctuating, thought disordered". We discussed what everyone was trying to do to no avail and then I agreed to make a complaint, this time to Victorian health authorities.

The VDDS, Victorian Dual Disability Service, should have been contacted much earlier by the Mental Health Unit. We tried to set that up even before Alex was transferred to Victoria. We kept reminding and they kept postponing.

4 August: So yet again I made another complaint, this time to the Regional Health Service and to the Victorian Mental Health Complaints Commission.

In summary:

- Alex needed urgent inpatient admission
- The Mental Health Unit for Small Town did not provide Alex enough support and did not refer him for inpatient admission
- The Mental Health Unit did not consider the urgency of Alex's situation.

Alex had been in Victoria one month and it was grim. If the complaints process could do anything it was not going to be in time for the urgent situation. The Commission began with a worry about needing Alex's permission to talk to me! I offered to send them the Guardianship Order. I emailed the Psychiatric Nurse at the Mental Health Unit again as follows:

> I despair.
> We are in a very dangerous situation with Alex. Staff are at serious risk.

Having only seen Alex asleep or drowsy this week for your assessment, I do not think you are taking this seriously if you do not listen to the observations of others.

You have been misled by Dhulwa to believe that Alex always hears voices. Yes he was reported to be hearing voices/paranoid in the period since January when he went through a florid psychosis post removal of antipsychotics and lithium because of the NMS. In that period the only resumption of antipsychotic was with clozapine. He was not hearing voices all last year and for other long periods of his life. He has not ALWAYS, as in he has not continuously, heard voices throughout his 40 years. I submit that it is only when he is not optimally medicated that he hears voices or relives earlier hallucinations with fixation.

Dhulwa was not interested in optimising Alex's mental health prior to discharge. That institution had a vested interest in informing you that this was Alex's normal or baseline/ as good as it gets!

In any case the hearing of the voices is not the only symptom on which I am basing my belief that he is manic at the moment. I am referring to all the speech patterns (rapid and rapid changes of topic), preoccupations, lack of adherence to regular eating and sleeping, irritability and aggression, shopping excesses, avoiding meds, laughing hysterically about a fantasy in the middle of another topic etc.

Putting aside for the moment the question of whether clozapine, although essential, is sufficient overall, the most pressing point is that he is taking less than half the prescribed dose of clozapine over several days and would be expected to be showing some symptoms. The fact that you do not recognise those symptoms as being due to mental illness is absurd.

Someone with ID and autism is going to exhibit mental illness symptoms consistent with those conditions. He is not going to all of a sudden show the same psychotic symptoms and ability to express his thoughts (usual and psychotic) as a person with normal intelligence.

I beg you to consider administering depot aripiprazole accepting any added risk of NMS re-emerging. The alternative seems to be solitary confinement in jail after someone is seriously hurt.

I have been leaving liaison to the Worker Support Organisation but I am prepared to not let this current situation rest. I will speak out where I see negligence even if due to lack of resources. I have been the carer of Alex for forty years, have a scientific background, and have made it my business to try to follow diagnoses and options for treatment all that time, as no other one single professional has ever shown consistent interest/ follow up or persistence to look broadly. It was always my efforts to seek out help. It is only very recently that his rare mutation was identified.

Please listen to me.

This produced no reaction. No help.

Other psychiatric advice must be available

The Support Coordinator and I continued a search for an independent psychiatric assessment, ideally from someone with qualifications in intellectual disability psychiatry. I identified a psychiatry practice in the region with a dual expert, thinking he could be an advisor but this was a dead-end. Alex was not accepted there with the excuse that he would need emergency services that they did not provide. This practice would not countenance being a consultant advisor to the Mental Health Unit for Small Town. There are many systemic issues that thwart proper care for those with intellectual disability and mental illness. I did internet searches and made a list. I eventually found a dual-disability psychiatrist who was willing and for whom the Support Coordinator applied for Victorian Multiple and Complex Needs Initiative (MACNI) funding.

5 August – Another Mental Health Unit Review with the Psychiatric Nurse who reported to the community Care Team that for 45 minutes Alex was drowsy due to lack of sleep the previous night, and had engaged in conversation. A call was made from Dr O to the Behaviour Specialist regarding the complaint made to the Mental Health Commissioner. Were they taking it seriously?

10 August – The Care Team tried to develop constructive connections. The Director of the Behaviour Specialist Organisation and the Support Coordinator met with the Sergeant and 2 senior constables at Small Town Police Station to discuss ongoing collaboration. They thought they left this meeting with an understanding.

A family gathering against the odds

14 August – Alex's big fortieth birthday. I had put a lot into planning this party not knowing whether we could go through with it. Extended family members were great in helping put it on. His closest friends from Canberra made the trip especially to wish him many returns: support workers and his nurse friend. We chose a community hall with lots of space outside for children (and separation from Alex if required) and a big kitchen from which we could serve food for lunch. We arranged for music and a biographical slide show. We decorated the hall. His aunt arranged for a magnificent cake. It was the first and only occasion Alex met his nephew, Miles.

Alex arrived in the costume he wanted but was late and did not want to leave when our rental of the hall was supposed to finish. He was so late, some people had to leave before he arrived. We managed to sing Happy Birthday and blow out candles. When he saw the groups were dwindling, he began to be upset. There were some stressful moments. Eventually we got him into the van to return to Small Town. Being incident free was a huge blessing. There was an incident the next day nonetheless.

Not looking good for Alex's future in Small Town

15 August – Dr O reviewed Alex while I was present at the house: Dr O greeted Alex while in his room and expressed the desire to speak to me. In the absence of agreement from Alex who was grumpy, Dr O instead took the two staff members to the front room to talk, leaving Alex alone in the living area with me. Alex became heightened over a technology issue and began an aggressive and rough episode against me. He pinned

me against the kitchen bench pinching my upper arms and grappled me with his arm about my neck and face. I called out for help but it was not for several minutes, and only with amplifying the call, did anyone come. I explained this was most unusual of Alex but Dr O appeared not convinced that Alex's behaviour was out of the ordinary. There was still no awareness that medical help was needed. Dr O called the police even though I was fine and Alex let me go. The police came to the house but went away satisfied that no further action on their part was required.

The Director of the Behaviour Specialist Organisation met with Dr O and others from the Regional Health Service. This meeting was marked for the differences in professional opinion displayed, with Dr O adamant that Alex was not manic. Dr O was not listening to me and not listening to experienced professionals. We requested the referral to VDDS (the Victorian dual disability service) again.

18 August – Care Team Meeting – we discussed the lack of medical help: Dr O noted manic symptoms now but as a stress response. I had defended my disagreement by telling him that such behaviour had been persistent since the removal of clozapine and aripiprazole early in his admission to the Adult Mental Health Unit late 2017 and despite use of olanzapine and then risperidone throughout 2018. In the absence of antipsychotic medication, the first symptoms to emerge were mania and paranoia. Clozapine and depot aripiprazole were again removed because of the NMS in January 2022 and whilst clozapine was resumed, the mania had persisted and was ignored so that he would be eligible for discharge. There was a period during which Alex was without mania which was 2021

when he was treated with lithium as well as the antipsychotics. He was no less stressed, being a resident of Dhulwa at this time.

The police reported an incident at the Small Town corner store (IGA) in which a young boy had been terrified of Alex who had supposed the boy gave him a disparaging look. The IGA subsequently banned Alex from visiting the shop.

Dr O and Registrar (unnamed) were to conduct the fortnightly review of Alex. The Psychiatric Nurse confirmed a reference to requesting referral to VDDS reflected in Dr O's notes. The Sergeant (Small Town Police) called Alice, the Support Worker Coordinator, highlighting community discontent at Alex remaining under the Mental Health Unit, and recommended that Alex be "moved back to Canberra, or will require sectioning under Mental Health Act". There was also an email to the Building Developer of the SDA from Small Town police, expressing concerns around Alex's suitability for their community in the light of recent incidents.

22 August – There was a meeting of the Care Team with the SDA developers to consider police complaints and modifications that might make the facility more secure, and thus increase confidence of Small Town townspeople. The developers were concerned about the effect on other disability residents of all the negativity to Alex in addition to the injustice to Alex of the current reactions. There was no legal basis to deny the facility as a place of residence for Alex.

23 August – An email was sent from the Behaviour Specialist to the police, advising them of relevant services in Alex's care,

and that the SDA developer was not an appropriate method of communication regarding Alex.

25 August – Care Team Meeting – Discussed a new incident on highway– Police closed off part of the highway and Alex had returned home by time of the meeting (2:30pm).

26 August – I made a call to the Mental Health Unit, concerned that Alex's behaviour was deteriorating. Psychiatric Nurse – Case Manager answered and stated he thought **the situation was overall positive and that the upsets were entirely understandable given Alex's big move from the ACT to a foreign place with so many new faces in Victoria.**

They were living in a separate universe! What hope did any of us caring for Alex have to get access to medical care for him?!

31 August – I attempted to take Alex to attend an ophthalmologist appointment in preparation for a cataract operation in his right eye. Alex spent his time from alighting the transport vehicle to final departure (which was about two hours) trying to make friends with anybody and everybody with inappropriate advances and physical contact. He was not able to see the specialist because he got heightened and aggressive when the oculist shone a light into his eye before he could even see the specialist. Alex was brought to the attention of the facility and security. He was really difficult about returning to the vehicle but fortunately he was taken home before police attended. Police were called by a member of the public it seems. He cannot keep appointments until his manic symptoms are addressed!

1 September – Care team meeting: team members agreed that Alex was mentally ill even if doctors could not see this and his behaviours were not going to improve under the current

treatments so we needed to cancel all his physical health appointments. There was a clozapine-required blood test soon which might be at risk. We still had no confirmation that Dr O had anything useful from VDDS.

When we did hear about VDDS a couple of days later, the report was they advised Dr O to continue as he was, but Dr O had not told them the full story and certainly not of the most recent events and list of manic symptoms!

The disability worker Shift Notes reflect:
- Day shift Alex very heightened, some self-harm and confronting in the neighbourhood, banging on doors, getting angry with yelling altercation with neighbours: one of the neighbours called the police. Coordinator spoke on the phone for some time with Alex and eventually had him return home.
- PM shift had sleep in afternoon but spent time heightened in evening yelling and screaming at staff.
- Night shift noted Alex screaming, slamming doors and asking staff to get out of his house. Staff attempted to redirect Alex to try calming Alex down, nothing seemed to have worked. Alex remains awake throughout the night playing music very loud, laughing and dancing. Alex was heard making threatening remark to staff saying "I am going to slit your throats with the bread knife".

Alex had never hurt anyone in this fashion and it was difficult to assess his intentions with such threatening language.

There was also a call from the Sergeant at Small Town to the Behaviour Specialist – He said he "can't guarantee Alex's safety in the community – threats from community members to 'take matters into their own hands' and threats to 'hit Alex with a baseball bat'".

2 September – (Friday) I spoke with a senior member of the Support Worker Organisation, very concerned that the weekend was commencing with Alex in a bad state and there was no health help available. That lady rang her superior later in the afternoon in between calls with the staff to manage the incidents occurring with Alex and asked if she should call the mental health team. The superior responded that she could, but that the last couple of times they had called leading into the weekend, the service had just simply said that there is nothing they can do and that the support workers should call emergency services if Alex is a risk to others. Of course, this was not going to be helpful as the Regional Hospital had declared it would not take Alex.

Then Alex's time in Small Town came to an abrupt end.

Unprecedented rage

3 September – There was the notorious incident at home in the evening with damage to property, including staff cars, harm to self and terrorising staff. Alex was capsicum sprayed and taken by police to the Regional Hospital. The office equipment was damaged beyond repair. The house was damaged badly and was assessed by staff as uninhabitable.

What happened that night? As indicated by the previous days' reports, Alex was most unwell. Each day was worse than before, with police involved and increasing concern from neighbours. No mental health support was given. Alex made threats against his workers in his heightened state. He had done this sort of thing to nurses at Dhulwa and had never carried it through. This Saturday night he again made threats, this time to cut their throats. He mostly wanted to sound tough as he had seen in the movies, but this was spine-chilling. Any knives were of a safety variety meaning they were not very sharp and had no dagger end. That does not mean they were harmless. One of the workers confiscated Alex's kitchen knives when Alex was not looking, as a safety precaution, but this exacerbated Alex's rage and he became destructive. How did they keep going with no help from health services?

Alex's moods that day escalated to a new high. In keeping with Alex's usual sensitive approach to his possessions, when he discovered the knives were missing, he regarded it as a big infringement of his rights. With his mental state at the time, he went into a blind rage. He damaged a lot of property including the workers' cars but he did not physically connect with the workers to hurt them. He damaged the staff phone so communication to the organisation and to me was delayed. I do not know who rang the police.

There was extensive damage to the house, most noticeably to a front window and the front door but throughout several rooms. Police arranged for hoarding to secure the house. The subsequent repair of the house that I took responsibility for was a long saga of residual angst against me as Alex's mother, which was an agony for me, but it was also part of why Alex was then homeless and this contributed to his decline.

The discharge had been set up for failure. As discussed in Chapter 10, I suspected that Dhulwa gave insufficient or misleading information to the Regional Health Service along the lines of discharging Alex as no longer psychotic, so it was up to community services to manage his intellectual disability-induced behaviours. I was not listened to by the Mental Health Unit. The Mental Health Unit psychiatrist used the competencies of the Support Worker Organisation in holding things together thus far as confirmation that Alex was not mentally ill! How jinxed can you be?

There were to be even deeper chambers to the hell Alex was in after two months in Victoria. Further frustration and decline commenced with the next ten days in the Regional Hospital which acted consistently with its declaration that it would never take him.

Chapter 12 Too little, too late
September 2022

Details of each of the next health services with responsibility for Alex is warranted in understanding the continuing decline. The first Victorian Mental Health Unit service was remiss but the Regional Hospital was appalling. From the Regional Hospital the story progresses to inadequacies in the Northern Health Mental Health Unit, Melbourne and thence in the Western Melbourne Mental Health Clinic.

Alex was taken to the Regional Hospital by ambulance on Saturday night, 3 September 2022 after the police attended the house in Small Town. This hospital behaved as if he had no rights to health services. They wanted him shunted anywhere else as soon as possible. The hospital premise was that he had disabilities separately from any mental illness and these were the cause of his bad behaviours. According to the Regional Hospital, these behaviours were not being managed as they should by his carers, who should have taken more responsibility, and not dumped Alex at the hospital.

The hospital, supposedly, did psychiatric assessments and concluded he was not showing any mental illness. If the psychiatric staff approached Alex without understanding his other disabilities, then I expect they asked him questions such as "how is your mood?', "Have you been seeing things?" and "Do you know what day it is?". Alex had always wanted to say he was not ill so he would just answer such questions with positive words such as I am fine. Alex would often know exactly the date, time, place and person he was talking to when he was manic and paranoid. Being so oriented does not preclude these symptoms. Alex was heavily sedated on arrival so I do not know when they did these nominal assessments. And why did they not speak to me, his guardian?

The inappropriate behaviours from the Regional Health Service included:

- contacting other organisations seeking advice on their capacity to provide community support for Alex, without my consent
- continued pressure on the community team, to remove Alex from the Emergency Department despite high level negotiations occurring throughout
- rude treatment of Alex's team, particularly of the Support Coordinator
- information insecurity –in sharing Alex's information with external organisations and with an individual (my landlord), and
- excluding me from email trails and in general not showing willingness to work with me.

The Support Workers had not been able to call me on the night of 3 September because their phone was broken. On Sunday 4 September I found out what had happened when a doctor rang me at 2 am from the Emergency Department. I was told

Alex was heavily sedated so I focussed on the insecurity of the house with its reported smashed front window and front door. I was able through various contacts to get someone for repairs to come the following day (Monday).

On Sunday I received calls from hospital staff such as the emergency social worker. There ensued a ridiculous series of calls in which I was told by the hospital that the Support Worker Organisation said something which I knew to be untrue. I felt as if they were playing games with a desire to make out a case against the Support Worker Organisation. I was told that the workers had abandoned Alex. There had been a communication problem with the newly created out of hours line for the support worker organisation, but I was able to give the hospital an alternative number. I told the hospital representative, that we needed to have conference calls so that the story was the same between all parties.

The hospital was not going to officially admit Alex but found him a bed in a mental health assessment area. They were able to assign minimal nursing staff with the support workers coming in 24/7 – far from abandoning Alex.

The NDIS Crisis Team became involved, and they too adopted the line that Alex's Support Worker Organisation was the problem. This attitude was so widespread at this stage that I wondered, when I also heard Small Town residents were saying the same thing, if the idea of confidentiality of information was non-existent. They were all talking to one another freely and it seemed as if the police were the connection between the hospital, my landlord and the rest of the Small Town community.

House damage complications

The real estate agent rang me wanting an account of the damage. I had thought I would have to wait until Monday to contact them so had not tried that day. The parents of the owner of the house lived in the same street and had heard, or witnessed, the incident on Saturday night, informing their son, my landlord. I explained to the agent what I was doing about rectifying the damage but I had not seen it for myself at that stage. The agent said the owner was not angry but did not want Alex living there anymore. I assured the agent that Alex would not return to the house. I had spoken to the agent on 1 September listing some damage that had occurred at that stage, promising repairs. The call on 1 September was based on the landlord receiving a letter about damage from the police. What were the Small Town police doing?

Hospital behaving badly

At 3:50 pm there was a teleconference attended by the NDIS Crisis Team, an emergency social worker from the Regional Hospital, Behaviour Specialist and management from the Support Worker Organisation as well as me and my daughter-in-law. We explained the challenges of trying to manage Alex in the community when the true state of his mental health was only discovered once he was *in* the community. The social worker said that the hospital Psychiatrist had cleared Alex of any mental illness but if we had any information that was important about his baseline etc., she would appreciate it. *Really? Why had they not asked for it?*

Alex's Behaviour Specialist explained the clear difference of professional opinion between him and Dr O, namely that Dr O thought Alex was in behavioural distress. However, the Behavioural Specialist said Alex's continued periods of heightened states was not consistent with this theory. When the social worker commented again about their psychiatrists being able to make assessments only on what they saw, both I and my daughter-in-law interjected about how they should have asked me for the background and context!

The Behaviour Specialist did not mince words given the treatment we had received. Alex had significant mental illness and it definitely was not because of social convenience that he was taken to hospital which had been the accusation. We spelt out the risks of placing him in the community without considering the reality of his illness. We were dealing with more than an accommodation issue. The social worker said she had to consult higher management.

5 September – Monday. Behaviour Specialist met with the Regional Health Service along with the After Hours Crisis Response (AHCR) Team, which is an external contract held by Marathon Health. External house damage was fixed and house made secure again. The police had arranged hoarding but the repairs were essential for the sake of the owner in my view.

Liaison continued between the Support Worker Organisation, Support Coordinator, and Behaviour Specialist throughout the day regarding details from a meeting held the previous day. Support Coordinator had not been in attendance as it was a Sunday. The agenda covered any potential alternate properties for Alex, feedback for the hospital regarding mental health presentation and information of fluctuation in Alex's state over prior 8 weeks.

Then the Nurse Unit Manager – Emergency – advised that the Emergency Department was likely to discharge Alex to 'Quest Apartments' with 2:1 Alex's own support workers. The shunting of Alex back in the community without any treatment was frightening.

Unequivocal statements but advice ignored

My daughter-in-law and I sent an email to the Liaison officer at the Regional Health Service including the following:

> **We are concerned that Alex is demonstrating signs of a manic relapse, possibly with psychotic features. We have observed signs of this relapse, since Alex was taken off lithium and additional antipsychotic in February this year after developing NMS. Alex has mostly definitely not been at his baseline since then. His mental health continues to deteriorate since his move to Victoria from Canberra.**

> Signs that his family and his NDIS support workers have noted include:
> - **Mood swings, increased mood lability.** Alex's mood rapidly shifts between elation, irritability and anger with no discernible trigger. His ability to tolerate frustration or change is non-existent. This is not in keeping with his baseline. Alex's normally tolerates changes of plans, different ideas reasonably well, and his frustration is relatively predictable. He will, when well, stick to his ideas, plans and routines, and can get frustrated if someone insists on another idea, but not to this extreme, or level or irrationality.
> - **Increased goal directed activity**: Alex's is pursuing activities to a bizarre and disorganised degree. He does usually have obsessional interests (photography, DVD,

scanning photos, art) that he pursues in a fixated and determined manner. However, his current disorganised, impulsive behaviour is not usual for him when he is well.
- **Delusional, grandiose and persecutory ideas and delusional misinterpretation:** Alex has been consistently voicing to family and carers grandiose and persecutory ideas. Recent examples of this include that he was the president, and recently he left a voicemail on Helen's phone saying gangsters had broken into his home and there was blood everywhere. When Alex becomes psychiatrically unwell he interprets normal things with delusional overlay (e.g. the home alone movie which he has always loved for its humour, he begins to think is real and believes either he is a gangster, he is part of the film or gangsters are after him). He also believes that people who may glance at him, are calling him names e.g. spastic, retard, and believes cars driving past are calling out insults to him.
- **Insomnia:** Very limited sleep.
- **Disorganised behaviour:** Alex ability to complete a task has deteriorated, he stops and starts things, goes off on tangents and is unable to complete tasks that were previously routine to him
- **Disorganised thoughts:** Alex's thoughts jump about in conversation, he goes off on odd, unrelated tangents and returns to odd persecutory and grandiose ideas. This is not typical for him.
- **Disinhibited interpersonal behaviour and over-familiarity:** Alex's interpersonal interactions are vastly altered, he is quick to anger at people with no perceived trigger and is often inappropriately familiar (e.g. asking neighbours over for cups of tea) which is not normal for Alex

- **Irritable and aggressive behaviour**: As mentioned, Alex's severity of anger, and violence is highly suggestive of him becoming unwell, it is not normal for Alex to behave in such an extreme way.

As we understand it, the mental health service thinks that the above behaviours are due to stress, intermittent medication non-compliance and the impact of his move to Victoria. We do not think that stress can account for the above presentation. Stress, his move, poor sleep and medication non-adherence may worsen his mental state, and can be contributing factors to his mental decline, but we do not think these are sole explanations for his presentation.

Risks that are currently occurring:
- A watch and wait approach, with some addition of PRN and a hope that Alex 'adjusts' to life is currently being adopted
- This is insufficient, and neglectful and does not appear to be cognisant of the risks and damage that are occurring of leaving Alex in such a volatile and unwell state.

Risks
- **Housing**: Alex has now damaged his house to the point where he is unable to be cared for safely in it
- **Financial**: Helen is now liable to pay thousands of dollars to repair the damage that has been caused, she is spending thousands on accommodation and travel in order to obtain short term accommodation to support Alex while he is so unwell
- **Reputational**: Alex has a permanent home in Small Town. His active psychiatric issues have led to him being banned from several areas (GP surgery, IGA) and many in the

community fearing him. This is extremely sad and unnecessary and contributes to Alex's feeling of isolation and being different.
- **Forensic:** There is a significant risk Alex will be arrested and incarcerated for actions undertaken while he is psychotic and his mood dysregulated.
- **Risks to others:** There is significant risk of Alex acting in a violent and impulsive manner to others while unwell.
- **Medical risks:** Alex has unable to get his routine dental care, ophthalmology care and GP care as he is too unwell to attend an appointment. He currently has un-investigated visual changes – it is not to be underestimated how significant the risk to his physical health is while his mental health issues are so active.
- **Psychiatric:** Alex's mental illness symptoms appear to go unrecognised and untreated by health professionals, and this prolonged period of under-treatment may impact his ability to return to his known baseline of recovery.
- **Quality of life:** Alex's general QOL is very poor, he is so agitated and disorganised he is unable to make new friends, complete his activities that he loves (e.g. art, photography), see his family in a calm and meaningful way.
- **Discrimination:** Alex appears to be discriminated against due to his disability. Family and In Life (his NDIS support team) have been told that "the large Regional mental health unit will never admit Alex". The message that this sends to us is that they are not prepared to provide mental health care for him, we believe this violates his basic rights to health care. The family and his support organisation asked for a referral to VDDS before Alex even moved to Victoria, it appears there is great reluctance for this, and this only occurred a week or so ago at great insistence. We don't know why there would be reluctance for this.

The message that we have received via social workers and ED staff is that Alex does not have mental health issues and there is no acute issue to be addressed.

- We, his family, and community disability professionals dispute that
- We ask for this to be reconsidered
- If Alex is discharged without these issues being addressed then there is very likely going to be a repeat of the circumstances that brought him in to hospital

Requests:
- Reassessment of Alex for consideration of a psychiatric admission, to re-examine him for signs of mental illness and consider the collateral history from family and from his professional community contacts (e.g. behavioural psychologist and NDIS support staff) who strongly believe that Alex is not at his baseline and is demonstrating signs of a relapse of his schizoaffective disorder
- Psychiatric admission to stabilise his mental state and consider optimising his psychotropic management of his schizoaffective disorder
- Consultation and family meeting with psychiatric staff who are making clinical decisions regarding his care to discuss with family their concerns about his mental state
- A comprehensive, longitudinal perspective, with a file review from past psychiatric assessments, interviews with family and community professionals, and involvement of VDDS occur to adequately assess Alex's mental health status

Could we have spelt it out more clearly? Did we need a megaphone to get anyone to listen? The Regional Hospital was not having anything to do with our requests.

Hospital ridding themselves of Alex regardless

Tuesday 6 September: The Support Coordinator was notified in a handover from the After Hours Crisis Response (AHCR) – and advised that Alex was ready for transfer, but the Support Worker Organisation was the barrier. Again, the hospital was keen to create this story even though the Support Worker Organisation was providing in-hospital support workers at this time, two per shift. The hospital was also not taking into account the problems with finding appropriate accommodation for Alex who could no longer live in the uninhabitable rental house. Never mind his mental illness too!

The Support Worker Organisation advised that the Quest apartments were unsuitable to Alex's disability needs, and they could not provide support in such an environment due to the risk to Alex, Staff and Community.

The hospital requested a new provider be engaged, and provided options, but the Support Coordinator advised this decision should be made by the nominee (guardian) and reiterated the importance of Alex's care model, the significant time it would take to establish a care team, the training which had to occur, all of which was not a quick solution. Further, we argued that a robust environment is integral to meeting Alex's needs at that stage.

The Support Coordinator obtained information about a single bedroom robust unit available in Northern Melbourne. The

Director of Social Work spoke of another option of an 'unused sub-acute setting' for Alex to move to with his Support Workers, and clarified the Regional Health Service would not provide any further involvement. The Care Team discussion would commence the next day regarding the viability of both options, and would hold a meeting with the Department for Families, Fairness and Housing (DFFH) Intensive Support Team (IST).

The Director of Social Work, Regional Health Service, contacted a local support provider at executive Level, to see if they had capacity to provide support and housing with Alex. This was done with no prior consultation with me or the team, done with no appreciation of the necessity to retain his current support workers and to not introduce a whole new organisation and workers who would have to start learning about Alex anew. The messages about what was seen as best for Alex continued to be at cross purposes. I requested that the Director of Social Work remove any prospective new provider from the email thread, due to privacy concerns because of information given therein. They had been so keen to engage their chosen provider that they forgot Alex's privacy.

The Support Coordinator and Behaviour Specialist met with the Department of Fairness, Families and Housing Intensive Support Team, who requested a timeline of Alex's time in Victoria and would consult with Office of the Chief Psychiatrist.

The Support Coordinator provided in an email to the NDIA Complex Planner an update of events and notified the social worker that the Intensive Support Team had been consulted, and no further information could be provided at present.

Dr O contacted me and requested an update on whether Alex could return to Small Town yet. I advised him of the house damage and that a return would not be able to occur. We discussed the reported notion that support workers had dropped Alex at the Regional Hospital as they 'wanted a rest' – I requested a meeting with all parties involved. The social worker from the Emergency Department contacted me via phone and requested attendance at the video meeting on Thursday 8 September 9:30am to discuss a plan moving forward.

Moving into the fourth day since the Small Town incident, despite friction between the Regional Health Service and the community team, operations continued.

From 6-9 September, there were multiple emails into which the Support Coordinator had copied me, as Alex's guardian, but the Regional Health Service removed me from their responses.

Wednesday 7 September: The Director of Social Work called the Support Coordinator to tell him that my preference was maintaining Alex's existing support workers, but that I would be very willing for their named local support provider to be involved in Alex's care. They also advised that medication changes were imminent but did not clarify details. *Could this be for something better?*

She also advised that the Behaviour Specialist Organisation strategies were ineffective, and the opportunity for Alex to move into the new provider property was arranged. The Support Coordinator was not made aware that this was in Northern Melbourne which is 1.5 hours by car from Small Town and would require transfer to a new Mental Health Service. Liaison was arranged between the Behaviour Specialist, Support Worker Organisation, and Support Coordinator on the viability of using the existing support service in Northern Melbourne, due to staff travel from Western Melbourne or Western Victoria regional area.

I raised concerns that a risk assessment had not been conducted on the property regarding the safety of Alex, staff and community. I complained of the discrimination against Alex. Dr O defended the health actions as non-discriminatory, but I had explained to him that failure to take into account the differences in meaning of presentation for someone with a cognitive disability for decisions about psychiatric care was negative discrimination in providing access to care.

The Behaviour Specialist and Support Coordinator had productive meetings with the Intensive Support Team of the Department of Fairness, Families and Housing who was escalating concerns to the Office of the Chief Psychiatrist to liaise with the Regional Health Service. The Behaviour Specialist was also in contact with the Support Worker Organisation to put some support around staff messaging to Alex while he was in hospital, so there could be consistent and reassuring messages. The Behaviour Specialist was planning to do the risk assessment of the proposed property but could see that Alex was not going to be any better at a new community location if they were not going to address his mental illness. Alex's community team was very concerned. Now I had the kind of team support I had been wanting for a while but we were up against a bigger machine than in the ACT.

On Thursday 8 September at 9.30 am the Regional Hospital held a family meeting at their request, with Dr O, the Director of Emergency and the Director of Social Work with me and my daughter-in-law also in attendance. The unsuitability of the Regional Hospital for Alex was set out. They were concerned that someone who did not need health care, in their assessment, might stay!

The potential involvement of the proposed new provider was reported. Again, the behaviour strategies used to date with Alex were claimed to be inadequate, minimising whether he had a mental health issue to be dealt with. I emphasised the need for something different in his medical care otherwise he could not live in the community. I stated that use of current supports is essential.

Redirection to the medical urgency

They began again talking about the urgency of doing something. I was losing patience and told them I was glad they recognised the urgency. I wanted to make sure we all appreciated the urgency. There was work being urgently done about the accommodation. The doctor needed to also do something urgently. I turned to him and asked when he was going to do something. Was he going to wait until Alex seriously hurt someone before he would act? He looked at me, or seemed to in this video meeting, as if he heard, but he had no answer.

This aversion to seeing the medical needs of someone with cognitive disability is compounded when the problem is mental illness, when the symptoms can be brushed away as due to disability and not due to treatable conditions.

I advised the Regional Health Service that the Northern Melbourne property was to be reviewed by the Behaviour Specialist for a Risk Assessment. The response email requested bringing this forward. The Behaviour Specialist sent a detailed email to the team providing the review of the property.

The DFFH IST requested a full discharge meeting, and offered to attend. This was never conducted. IST was informed of escalation to the Office of the Chief Psychiatrist (OCP) which requested no further move towards discharge without consultation from OCP and a robust-discharge plan, including meeting held with IST representatives.

I visited Alex which I had been doing daily once he was less sedated. He was asleep again and his workers were in a staff meeting. I waited up the corridor. At one stage I crept up to Alex's room to see how he was and went back to my seat after seeing him still asleep. The next thing a nurse appeared at my elbow, saying "I have to ask you to leave. The support workers are not present". I went towards the door then stopped. I was sick of people who made me feel bad when I was just going about my business with good intentions. I told her she was being officious with those words to which she replied that she thought she was being polite.

Just at that moment Dr O appeared asking to speak to me. He sat me down in a consultation room and I admitted I was tired.

He said that he had re-considered and perhaps indeed Alex was showing something of those symptoms I had spoken of. I wondered what brought that change of attitude!

Revolution!! He would prescribe a new antipsychotic better directed against manic symptoms, cariprazine. It worked via much the same mechanism as the medicine that I kept saying worked with Alex, aripiprazole. He would start Alex on a very low dose. He would also give Alex something else as an anticonvulsant, clonazepam, but not as a replacement for valproate.

I remember saying at some stage in this interview with Dr O that I was not worrying about his physical health at the moment. In retrospect this seems like words that should haunt me. I did not mean I was happy for him to have only a few months to live. I was thinking more about how we needed him in a better mental health state before any action for his physical health could be achieved.

My struggles as carer

I was not feeling well and tested positive for COVID 19 the next day. I must have been half asleep when Dr O told me about the cariprazine. I had not asked Dr O whether he would increase the dose and at what rate. What was his plan? What was his consideration of the potential for NMS to occur again? I supposed he would be professional about the ongoing care! Alas! There is no system but chaos for someone moving from one mental health unit to another in Victoria. That was the last I heard from Dr O. What was his handover regarding his patient starting a new medicine and any advice about monitoring for either positive effects or negative side effects?

And the Regional Hospital did not even tell his next mental health unit that Alex was now on cariprazine.

The Regional Hospital staff gave me a hard time. Was it deliberate? Because I had a son with problems there, did that mean I needed to be oppressed? I mentioned the nursing staff above kicking me out one day. I also had to suffer three security guards descending on me on one of my visits to Alex. They took me aside to be searched! I had brought Alex a pencil case with drawing and writing pens and pencils a day or so earlier. I only noticed when I took the pencil case into the ward that Alex had secreted a small knife into it before the trip to hospital. This was a round ended knife but nonetheless I brought it to the attention of the nursing staff who kept it and gave it back to me on my way out. The security guards now pronounced me a threat because I dared bring a knife to the ward, even if unknowingly. I told them I would cooperate but what they were doing was silly given what actually happened. One of the guards began to be a bit embarrassed when I gave details but the boss guard was not to be deterred from protecting the facility from the menace I represented.

I had reason to question the attitude of staff early on, when I had the following encounter from someone manning the enquiry desk in Emergency. She was at the window where I had been directed to ask to enter the area where Alex was held and where I had been met with friendliness before. This new lady said I would have to go through another entrance and round the back. I tried to follow her directions and she came through to where I ended up, perhaps to check on me. A staff member there said I had come the wrong way which annoyed the reception lady. I retraced my steps and managed to get in to Alex. The next day the same reception lady tried to redirect me in the same way. I said no, we did that yesterday. I said, "How about I ring Alex's nurses' station myself?" This worked. She came through to Alex's area to check up on this breach of her guard against nuisance parents. Did they not even consider that my life was in considerable distress and my son needed me to be functional?

I was out of action with COVID-19 for most of the next week and only have a sketchy idea of what happened while I was in isolation. I could not help with Alex's packing and his move but could attend to communications with the team through my phone or lap-top. Fortunately, I had already engaged a repair person for the internal damage to the house but I could not inspect the works for a while.

Also on this day, the Mental Health Unit for Small Town called the Support Coordinator to request an update on Alex's whereabouts and plan for handover to another mental health service. I do not know if it happened.

On 9 September Friday, the seventh day in the Regional Hospital, I was contacted by a third social worker from the hospital regarding my consent for training to commence with the proposed new provider. I did not consent as none of us were clear on what training was being referenced, or why the provider was involved. There were issues with information security again here.

How not to handle a discharge

The DFFH IST met with the Regional Health Service and advised that there existed a list of requirements prior to discharge but this was not shown to anyone in the team. The social worker of the Emergency Department contacted the Support Coordinator asking what time discharge would take place, on that day. The Support Coordinator advised of high level discussions and that the discharge would NOT be taking place that day. There were multiple emails regarding my requests in relation to discharge; medications, treatment sheet, etc. I remain doubtful that any of them were provided given the way the new mental health unit reacted.

The Access and Resource Team at the Regional Health Service advised via email that the Clinical Director – Mental Health had liaised with the Office of the Chief Psychiatrist overnight, who were satisfied with the approach of the Health Service and therefore would be proceeding with discharge plans. Was this the recognition of the addition of cariprazine? Nothing more was explained.

The Support Coordinator specifically requested a handover from the Regional Health Service to Northern Health, in alignment with my request. This was not conducted it seems, as the Northern Health Mental Health Unit cited issues, reported an insufficient handover and put through a Risk Notification (RiskMan) some weeks later to whatever authorities could act. The Northern Mental Health Unit said that there was an absence of critical information in the handover, and noted this was likely missed as a standard referral process had not been conducted. They complained that there was no transition plan, no mention of VDDS and being misled by the transfer being described as 'caretaker request' to the Northern Mental Health Unit. That is, the Northern Mental Health Unit was not aware of the level of consideration required of Alex as a complex case including observations associated with a new medicine.

Arrangements for discharge and transfer of Alex were fraught and required steering by the community team. On Monday 12 September the Emergency social worker tried to direct the Support Coordinator to a discharge by close of business but the Support Coordinator advised that discharge planning was to be conducted with the Intensive Support Team. It would be unlikely to occur prior to Wednesday, due to staff training, alterations to property and MOU signing between the Support Worker Organisation and the managers of the Northern Melbourne property. Staff Training session 1 was subsequently completed, facilitated by the Behaviour Specialist regarding changes in environment, planning for Alex and staff safety support worker care team with additional facility staff who will be on site because it was a shared property.

On Tuesday 13 September transport was arranged via the Victorian Ambulance Patient Transport. Training Session 2 was completed. Changes to property as per risk assessment recommendations were completed. The Regional Hospital said it would provide Webster packs for Alex's meds. Then the hospital said it does not provide Webster packs, so arrangements were made to send scripts to a pharmacy readily accessible by Alice.

Alex was transferred via ambulance patient transport to Northern Melbourne on Wednesday 14 September. No scripts were sent to the pharmacy as promised: hospital said it will make up Webster packs. The hospital then said they do not do

Webster packs. Alice set up communication between the hospital and the community pharmacy. Was this the Regional Hospital organisation at its best!?

Expert advice

We had earlier asked a Victorian psychiatrist, with expertise in intellectual disability, to prepare a report guiding the diagnosis and treatment of Alex, funded through the MACNI. With the events of Alex being taken to the Regional Hospital and the need to find accommodation, I asked this doctor to provide a preliminary report from which I quote:

> Alex Cameron is 40-year-old single man who has a complex neurodevelopmental and neuropsychiatric history. He previously lived in the ACT and moved to Melbourne in early 2022. Alex was recently taken to the Regional Hospital Emergency Department with escalating aggressive and destructive behaviours. He was unable to return to his accommodation because the damage caused by Alex had left it uninhabitable and he was denied admission to the adult mental health inpatient unit because he was assessed as not having a mental illness.
>
> I have been commissioned by MACNI to conduct a comprehensive assessment. I have been contacted today (13 October 2022) informing me about the very temporary nature of Alex's accommodation and indicating that there are serious issues regarding Alex's behaviour in the community. In response to the urgency of current situation I am providing a preliminary assessment based on written information from Alex's family, and assessment letters from a NSW psychiatrist specialising in intellectual

disability who consulted on Alex. I agree with this doctor's assessment that Alex has either a schizoaffective disorder or bipolar disorder with psychotic symptoms. I have not included references but can provide these on request and the final report will contain references.

It is my opinion that it is highly likely that Alex is currently manic with psychotic symptoms.

After completing this report, I received an email from Alex's mother Helen providing further details raising serious concerns about Alex's risks to himself and others. In the township of Small Town Alex has been socially inappropriate, intrusive, loud, frightening and aggressive. He is not welcome in town and there is talk about a restraining order. Alex has chased a young boy who he thought was looking at him disparagingly and he "did things" to worry kindergarten staff. He is clearly a risk to himself and others. He should be referred immediately to the local mental health services or taken to the emergency department.

The Victorian dual-disability expert confirmed what we had feared all along, what I, in my layman's way, had been trying to tell the Mental Health Unit, and it was quite clear that Alex needed acute medical help. Medical help as she recommended by the expert was not available from the Regional Health Service which behaved so appallingly, and as it eventuated, the new area with respite accommodation and the subsequent second respite area never provided the level of care required. The rationale for not doing anything was the general defence of "not wanting to risk harm by interfering in his current regime". This was disgraceful denial of access to proper care because of Alex's cognitive problems.

We were now very dependent on dosing with cariprazine being successful, but the barriers included:

- No notification to the new mental health unit that it was prescribed
- And thus no transfer of any plan for increasing the dose above the started dose (let alone decreasing his clozapine dose), and
- Certainly no guidance on what monitoring should be done on positive effects and any negative effects, which was of particular concern given his contraction of NMS earlier in the year.

There was another set of barriers to Alex's progress. Because of his risky behaviours in Small Town and no allowance for seeing effective treatment for his mental health before being moved to another community situation, the response was to keep him even more locked up. Everyone was risk averse, not believing he could have improved mental health. This restriction was not really conducive for best mental health nor for best physical health.

Chapter 13 The threat of homelessness

September - November 2022

The fragile accommodation situation for Alex was a direct consequence of him not being treated earlier when there was medicine available to help him. We noticed an almost immediate change in Alex after a week on cariprazine, but accommodation issues could not be resolved easily. On 20 September the care team reported:

- Alex has been more settled over past 5 days; able to engage in discussion and receive feedback, escalations in behaviour have not been as erratic or escalated as quickly
- Medication compliance still fluctuating, but more consistent than prior to hospital presentation 2 weeks ago
- PRN (sedation) administered 2 x (Friday and Sunday Afternoon/Evening) – both instances correspondence with missed medication same morning.

Even with improvements in his aggression and the other behaviours of concern, Alex's overall situation was actually declining. He was heavily restricted compared to residing in Small Town. It was not easy to get any improved behaviours from Alex translated into a more normal community life.

There was a long road to get any formal plans and worker protocols changed to allow for reduced restrictions and greater participation. Workers were unnerved by some of his shocking behaviour and not always able to read his moods and states of being heightened. He felt imprisoned. Alex was getting very little exercise at this stage and with a high clozapine dose his carbohydrate consumption was excessive.

The Northern Mental Health Unit did not engage well with Alex on a personal level in his short stay in that area, let alone see his symptoms and physical state. When they eventually came to see him, it was earlier on the appointment day than stated so that I did not get there in time. I was told Dr P came with a mask and face shield which I felt was overkill at that stage of the pandemic. Dr P further alienated Alex by standing back as if afraid of him, and when Alex wanted to take photographs in his usual friendly but over-solicitous fashion, the situation got awkward and the doctor had to leave, aggravating Alex.

There was no discussion about the cariprazine. On questioning later, the clinic contact said she would ask the Mental Health Unit doctor but nothing happened except that the script was renewed – for the same start up dose. There was no rationalisation provided.

By the third week of October while in Northern Melbourne, the team was fortunately talking about a step-down in Alex's Behaviour Support Plan which would make it more likely he would be taken out on walks or other places in Northern Melbourne. Alex asked if he could see Mary Poppins at Her Majesty's Theatre after seeing it advertised on television for early 2023. I bought four tickets immediately hoping this would be something we could work towards and give Alex something to look forward to. Alex would attend with me and two workers. Alex had been keen on theatre for a long time. He had participated in an acting group post-school which had taken him on trips to Japan and one to India for competitions as described earlier.

We did not forget Alex's needs in terms of his physical health including his need for a GP and specialists. If Northern Melbourne was very temporary, local professionals there would be of limited help and we were not sure yet of being able to get Alex out of any accommodation for medical visits. After the Small Town GP banned Alex, the nearby Smaller Town GP agreed to take him, which sounded good if he were to return to Small Town, which we still planned to do. Smaller Town changed its mind, apparently after hearing the opinions of the first town, but this was after I had filled out forms and arranged for transfer of Alex's notes, which they refused to return when I needed them to go to his finally found GP in Western Melbourne.

At the end of October, the Support Worker Organisation changed their management of Alex' team by introducing a house leader able to spend a lot more time at Alex's house. Thus Serena was introduced into Alex's life for the better. Serena got to know Alex quickly and gained his trust.

Soon after, we realised that Alex would have to move house. There were no possible extensions because of the Northern Melbourne facility's commitments already in place. It was only ever made available as respite. The situation looked disastrous.

Was Small Town still an option?

Alex was still due to take up the original SDA offer in Small Town and we had hope he would be well enough on the new medicine. His reputation preceded any easy resumption of such plans in Small Town.

The townspeople were still in a rage and wanted to do anything to stop him returning. With the leakage of information rife, we assumed Small Town knew where he was and under what circumstances. Egged on by police, a town group, interested in progress on their terms, organised a town meeting on 12 October 2022. This meeting was nominally about 'town planning' but which became a meeting inviting release of rage about Alex. I was given reports of the meeting from those in Alex's community team able to be present. They said that the attendees aired personal and confidential information about Alex, which could only have come from loose-lipped professionals, including the number of days he was in the Regional Hospital and supposedly what his NDIS funding was. Some things presented as facts were inaccurate or wrong.

Some things talked about were supposedly from eye witnesses of the violent incident in Small Town of 3 September. The stories seemed to be from the frenzied imagination circulating in Small Town. For example, exaggerating Alex's violence towards workers when he wrecked support worker equipment and chased them but did not catch them and no one was injured.

The townspeople turned Alex's love of taking photographs into the accusation that he was a paedophile. His unbelted, ill-fitting pants worked against him, in that when he took photos using two hands, his pants fell down increasing willingness to think the worst of him. Alex was also particularly paranoid about children as the source of name calling and when ill, could show loud behaviour when he was near children. Furthermore, I heard that the townspeople got mixed up with someone who had been living in Small Town with the name Alex who had an unfortunate habit of dropping his pants.

I heard there was something in a local paper about Alex, perhaps a reader's letter, fanning the frenzy. I did not follow this up, as I expected it would be devastating to see it in print.

The people planned to have another meeting and set up a petition to the relevant Minister trying to prevent Alex living in Small Town. Not only did they decry Alex, but they put down his Support Worker Organisation. A fiction was spreading that the organisation did not know what they were doing. One of the letters put in mailboxes, from Alex's Support Workers during his time there, unfortunately highlighted autism inaccurately as an explanation for Alex. This was picked up by laypeople as the key for managing Alex without realising that Alex's mental illness symptoms needed to be treated first. I was not free to correct the misunderstandings without breaching Alex's confidentiality.

We had a meeting with the developers of the SDA on 15 October. Someone from the Shire Council joined in. The SDA developers' lives had been made difficult with the reactions from residents, the misjudged communications from police and the expressed opinions from others that the SDA building designs were wrong. Those focussed on development of Small Town were demanding assurances that Alex would be kept safely away from the people. We did not have much time before the 1 December finish line for the SDA. The SDA developers needed to be confident that Alex was taking up the offer.

A dreadful decision

I thought back to how we arrived at this situation. Despite the risks, we had all been led to believe by Dhulwa that Alex was suitable for discharge. The Support Worker Organisation and Behaviour Specialist were taken by surprise by Alex's state on arrival in Small Town. They had to act with no support from the Mental Health Unit and negativity from the Regional Hospital. They were caught out not giving information to neighbours because it was all so unexpected. They belatedly tried to reassure neighbours with letterbox drops to give an explanation and to give residents contact numbers if they were worried. In some cases, these letters only served to further frighten people. One cannot blame the residents for being scared, as Alex could get very loud, and with his big frame, look very aggressive. Some people were kind even if they were worried or scared. A couple of neighbours were actively helpful. My issue is with those Small Town residents who thought that Alex's behaviours meant he deserved to have his rights ignored.

In reality, all well Alex wanted and asked for was for others to be kind and to have friends. He strove to be good and a valued member of the community. When he was chastised as a child he would say "but I want to be good, Mum".

The lack of mental health care was not visible to neighbours and other residents. Apparently doctors and nurses are infallible. The health services got away with their inadequacies. All residents could see was Alex with support workers so they blamed these workers' strategies and practice. Residents were not aware that the support workers had actually done an extraordinary job in minimising the chaos and damage while faced with someone in a very bad mental state.

By the first week of November, I had to make a decision to withdraw Alex from the SDA in Small Town. My reasoning was based on the poor health services and the way in which his life would be made a misery by the reactions from townspeople. I was also worried there would be racial prejudice against his support workers whose ethnic origins included South Pacific, Africa and India. It was also important that Alex's situation did not make it difficult for the other intended residents of the SDA development. Further, the Regional Hospital refused to look after Alex resulting in no back up for support workers, should Alex be unwell again.

I discussed his rights with a disability lawyer who confirmed that neither the police nor others had any legal right to stop him living in the SDA dwelling. We had kept planning as if he would return to Small Town. I could have kept fighting but had to reconsider. I came to the decision to make Alex homeless after all we had been through to secure an SDA dwelling! We had spent some weeks scanning the SDA situation around

Victoria to see if an alternative could be found. We did not discover any easy answer and I was very worried that other SDA sites would also be with bad health services. I had added to Alex's risks for settling well in Victoria.

The prejudiced health services and the emotional reactions of Small Town both contributed to Alex's further decline in Victoria. I can hear Dr K saying again I told you so! "If ACT cannot look after Alex, how do you expect a small town to look after him?", which is what he said when told of the plans to move Alex to Victoria. Dr K did not understand that the Support Workers did not live in Small Town and the mental health service was based in a larger town near Small Town. It was a broad regional system.

I submitted an addendum to my complaint in July to the Victorian Mental Health Complaints Commission with the following on 10 November as follows.

1. A new medicine has been prescribed but at a point of transfer to a different health area (for respite) with
   a) no plan/handover from Dr O at Mental Health Unit for Small Town for subsequent monitoring for side effects, signs of effectiveness and potentially increasing the dose above the baseline tentative start; and
   b) the Regional Hospital giving an incorrect medicine list on discharge to the respite area, including omission completely of the new medicine.
2. The Regional Hospital personnel were difficult to deal with because they made up their minds that Alex was not brought there for treatment but for "social reasons". Is this what the Mental Health Unit told them? The hospital

provided a bed under sufferance and lots of nagging to have him removed and with no assessment and treatment for his mental illness. Social workers were rude, misrepresenting what other parties had said during negotiations and quipping to community carers at the time of discharge that they should not just 'drop him off next time'. Northern Health Mental Health Unit was appalled at the lack of proper handover to look after Alex with all his complex needs, including physical health needs. The Regional Hospital gave out information about my son to a non-family member who rang up – the landlord of the house that was damaged by my son while he was ill. This landlord has no right to be given personal and health information about my son! The total picture is of poor standards, disregard for patient privacy and discrimination against my son because of his intellectual disability.
3. Small Town Medical Clinic on seeing Alex ill in its surgery put energy into banning him as patient, including from telehealth, rather than into any notion of care to say, speak to the Mental Health Unit about what might be done to help him, or to arrange an ambulance to take him to obtain the much needed treatment! Is this Victoria's mental health system at its best? – A system in which private GPs sidestep care for one of their patients simply because it should be someone else's problem rather than part of the whole person they are supposed to care for?
4. The Victorian dual disability psychiatrist is performing a detailed assessment of my son. The preliminary report, on noting my son's presentation during July and August within community at Small Town, said he was manic and

was a danger to himself and the community and should be taken immediately to hospital preferably by ambulance. This contrasts with the conclusions of the Mental Health Unit to Small Town who associated my son's presentation with, variously, autism, adjustment to living in a new area or being in need of sleeping tablets, and we should just wait with the carers managing. This Mental Health Unit does not appear to suffer any loss of professional reputation from their poor treatment of my son: they blithely continue in ignorance of their devastating role in my son's life.

5. The Mental Health Unit and the Regional Health Service get off scot-free but the Support Worker Organisation, community care provider, has been blamed and has suffered a loss of reputation within Small Town, as if the carers were supposed to be able to control a severely mentally ill person who was repeatedly denied proper treatment.

6. The preventable disaster that is still unfolding for my son, and is directly related to ACT's and Victoria's negligent mental health services, is as follows:

- His accommodation issues are still in crisis. With the delay in his SDA until 1 December, he is threatened with not being able to stay in his current respite for the wait. Above that insecurity, it appears that Alex will not be able to live according to his rights in his SDA.
- His SDA is in Small Town where the police have been working to stop him living there. They have had a public meeting defaming Alex and managed 110 signatures to a petition which has gone to a Victorian state Minister - Child Protections and Family Services - Colin Brooks. The

rage in the community means that Alex will never be welcomed and he will pick up on the antagonism at a time when he craves contact and friends. There will be another public meeting soon. The medical clinic has banned him and refused to arrange a telehealth appointment. Alex is banned from the only supermarket, the IGA. People are going to walk away, point and make disparaging remarks if they see Alex in the community.
- The Chair of the Small Town progress group is demanding that the Support Worker Organisation elaborate how they will keep the community safe from Alex. We cannot tell this person, police or the community that Alex had untreated mental illness, and could be expected to be much better now, for reasons of privacy and the high risk that it will just confirm the view in their minds that he is totally dangerous. It is also questionable what private information should be given to people who will share and gossip.
- As much as it would be ideal never to go near Small Town again, Alex has nowhere else to go on 1 December unless another respite can be found (for a lengthy stay while we search for another SDA) and NDIA agrees to pay for it (an uphill battle if the Small Town SDA is ready).
- He is unable to obtain general dental and medical care as he cannot yet be confidently taken by carers to appointments. He needs regular care for a number of chronic conditions. He has a cataract which should be rectified and loose teeth requiring urgent treatment. Getting his regular clozapine monthly blood test was extremely difficult this month with people being too scared to approach him still.

My son is now suffering the severe consequences of the mental health system's discrimination based on his intellectual disability. He has had the financial loss through the need for moving interstate, for house repairs, loss of friend and family contact, restrictive environments and loss of reputation affecting his ability to live according to his rights and needs in the future. There is no hope that this will be resolved soon. I kept telling the Mental Health Unit for Small Town that my son was ill, setting out his symptoms and suggesting treatment, but I was ignored and ignored which prompted my original complaint to you. The community care organisation with qualifications and experience in this area were ignored. The SDA developer has been put in a very difficult situation after all their work in a much needed sector. We all pay; doctors and others excuse themselves, despite being given all the relevant information and alerts, on the cover-all basis that my son is a complex case.

I want you to know that while Alex is on a better path thanks to some action from Dr O eventually, enormous damage has been done, devastating for all associated.

I have sent similar comments to the ACT Health's Dhulwa Inquiry.

When I was contacted by the Complaints Commission, I asked for an apology from the Regional Hospital but I never received one. The person did say however, that what I had written was useful for their consideration of reforms required, for which they had other complaints to build a picture.

All this time I had been trying to make sure the rental house in Small Town was being restored to the same condition as it had been in when I commenced the lease. Except for my time coping with COVID 19 and for Alex's needs, I was at the house making sure the trades people were engaged and had completed work started on 5 September. Unfortunately, the landlord turned against me even though he could see I had promptly engaged trades people to restore the house and was going beyond the damage in some cases.

I will here set out the actions of the landlord that I had the misfortune to acquire, not just because he unnecessarily made my life a misery but because I suspected he was engaged with Small Town police in spreading stories and actively trying to stop Alex living in Small Town. The landlord was involved in the general negative responses from Small Town.

I met the landlord when he stopped at the house in the week after the incident before or after visiting his parents at the end of the street. On 5 September he seemed open and calm about what must have been a dreadful experience for him with his house. He could see that I already had the front of the house repaired. He seemed to accept that I was doing the repairs and had his interests in mind. His mother had been quick to visit the damaged house on 4 September, as was my son Clive who had come from Canberra to support me on my current trip, while on that day I was on the phone to all the parties mentioned. Clive invited her into the house to see the damage if she wanted. He and I wanted to be transparent about what was required and did not realise what was going to emerge with the landlord. The mother took photographs.

On one of his visits the landlord told me he did not mind if Alex came back to the house. Contrary to this, he had said through the Agent that he did not want Alex returning to the house. This was my first indication that the landlord could oscillate.

He declined my invitation to look around the house if he wished. He told me he had phoned the Regional Hospital the day after the incident out of concern for Alex and was told yes Alex was at the hospital and that he was alone. This was not good. I wanted to disengage with this man on being told that. I did not show my unrest.

I had given my phone number to the landlord in the interests of making sure we coordinated over anything to do with the house. He and I had a chat on 8 September and he messaged me with comments that he thought I had the repairs under control.

We kept missing each other's calls towards the end of September but he left an SMS on 2 October saying he was just asking about the repairs. I was not well enough with COVID-19 to keep engaging on these in this way.

I complained to the agent on 7 October about the landlord entering the property without giving me notice. He had entered on two occasions that I knew of: one to install outside lights on his own whim and one when there was my tradesman inside (date unknown). The landlord had tried to get the tradesperson at the house to do extra work at my expense on matters present prior to the lease and which had nothing to do with the damage to the house by Alex or me. This tradesperson reported to me that the landlord had a good look around the house in my absence.

At another visit, the landlord wanted to ask me questions about my vacating or keeping the lease. I said I thought I should talk about those matters with his Agent, whom he had employed.

I sent the Agent notification on 9 October of a breakage of the post at the hinge of the side gate installed by the landlord, such that it could over-swing in the wind and pull on the hinge fixation point.

The landlord sacked his Agent and acted for himself from 11 October.

I received formal notification from the Agent on 13 October that the landlord would act for himself, telling me the landlord would be in touch with me. He did not get in touch with me except later to say (albeit politely) that I seemed to have forgotten to pay the rent! I had paid the Agent in the absence of being given a different mechanism. After the landlord sent me a reminder message about paying the rent, I had to explain to the landlord that he needed to give me his bank details.

The landlord wondered why he did not get the rent but before checking with me, he went to Alex's Support Worker Organisation's offices in Western Victoria saying I owed him rent and he could not get in touch with me. They told him it was nothing to do with them, of course. I now realised he was not to be trusted. He had my phone number and of course he could contact me. *What skewed thinking would induce him to go to the Support Worker offices?*

On sending my information about the repairs by email to him on 26 October, the landlord wanted me to answer questions about dates and the extent of damage and how it occurred. I refused to answer, as this seemed like a probe into Alex and it was not relevant to my efforts to restore the house and not part of my obligations. I was already suspicious of his discussions with Small Town police.

Harassment from Small Town landlord

By SMS on 31 October the landlord indicated he wanted to visit the next day (Melbourne Cup Day) to have a look at the progress of repairs. I did not need him to come to tell me more work was required. I had already said the repairs were not complete. I said he was not giving me enough notice, having recently agreed he would give me a week's notice. He called me a liar about my lease application. He tried to say that the Act said he could come with short notice for repairs. He did not comprehend that this clause is for landlords doing/arranging urgent repairs, not for inspections. He was not doing the repairs. I was. I said it was not convenient on Cup Day but tried to be elastic on the seven days' requirement for notice and suggested the following day. This was not convenient for him. I made it quite clear that I did not want him entering on Cup Day and I heard nothing more from him that night.

Late in the afternoon of 1 November, the landlord and another man (possibly his father but not introduced to me) tried to enter the house. The landlord used his own key to open the front door and there ensued a standoff as I held the door with my foot and body as he kept trying to push his way in. Also in the house was my brother whom I asked to call the police. The landlord said a lot of nasty things and tried to make out a false case that he was not told of the damage, despite:

- His mother having photographs taken the day after the incident
- Me speaking to his agent on two occasions about damage
- Me sending the landlord the same written information as I had sent the Agent, who had said it was adequate communication on the matter, and
- It was disingenuous as he had refused entry on my invitation in that first week.

He said my tradesperson told him the work was finished so why am I saying it is not finished?

He mocked me for telling him, from my sense of duty, about the unusual orientation of the new border fence being put up coincidently in the back, telling me I must think I am a structural engineer. He mocked me for shaking while I tried to hold the door. He attacked me about my academic qualifications saying I am ALWAYS using my PhD over people. The application form probably asked for academic qualifications. He accused me of lying on my application bringing up some supposed denial of Alex being my adult son. I think he was not understanding the limitations of the online form which only gave me the word options of using child instead of friend or spouse. I do not remember enough of the form to know why I omitted Alex's birth date but it gave the landlord an opportunity to declare with scorn that I did not know my son's birth date.

The landlord spoke about Alex making the street unsafe, which seemed to be his justification for harassing me. I asked him if this treatment of me was all about him trying to take advantage of my family tragedy. More mockery. He said something like, "This, this is not a tragedy mate. A car accident in which someone gets killed is a tragedy".

The landlord poured further scorn on me about some boxes he could see down the passage way, saying I could not be working very hard as he had seen those boxes like that a few weeks ago. "You better get on with it", he told me. He told me I was an awful mother. "Your son was taken away by police in an ambulance and you couldn't even be here. You could not even visit him in hospital. I rang the hospital and they told me."

When the other man tried to say something I abruptly and curtly asked him who he was. I was told I was rude.

They eventually left. I collapsed in sobs.

When the police came, they could see my state. "Did he hurt you?" they asked. "No, he just tried to use force to get in the house and I have had more than my share of stress", I replied. These policemen were constructive – from a coastal town fortunately, not from Small Town whose station was closed on the public holiday. The landlord would not respond to their calls at first but eventually did. The police reported back to me saying they explained to him that we were trying to look after the house and in their work, they knew what a trashed house looked like so he should not be worried.

The landlord's lawyer acted for him to arrange an inspection date. I agreed to a visit from the landlord with his lawyer, from local Small Town, and arranged for a witness of my own to be there to support me. The story from there bordered on the absurd at times, with misinterpretations, irrelevant matters and efforts again to make me pay for things which had nothing to do with me.

The lawyer accused me of not wanting to talk about the damage points and not showing them where the repairs had not been done. It did not seem to occur to him that I had no photographs like he and the landlord had access to and that most repair work was done while I was not able to get to the house because of my COVID-19 infection. They wanted to see what damage had not been addressed. I could not remember the full extent of the damage once the repairs were largely done. It did not seem to occur to him that the reason for my saying more work needed to be done was because the work was not yet to completion standard, not because some spots had not been started.

They took exception to Alex's support workers being with him 24/7, saying a business had been set up contrary to the lease. The lawyer was supposedly familiar with the disability sector, but did not give thought to the need for things like white boards for the communication between the multiple shifts required. As if having a white board in what the landlord regarded as a bedroom was counter to the lease! I had told the Agent at the start of the lease that staff would be coming to the house when Alex was there and named the Support Worker Organisation. I asked the Agent whether I had to name each support worker to which he said no. In the event of Alex's stay no staff ever slept there: all night duties were active. Having disability or aged care workers visit a client's house, even if this occurs round the clock, is not setting up a business at the house.

The lawyer and landlord tried to interpret my intentions on scarce evidence and had no idea about how Alex's NMS, mental illness relapse, delays in the SDA build and poor medical care resulted in plans being changed. The landlord put on a show at the inspection about the old irregular ceiling painting in his kitchen-family room, exactly as he had tried with the tradesperson working on the house, at the time he entered without notice to me. I told him it was nothing to do with me, that he could view the start of lease photographs and no, I was not going to pay half to re-paint. He kept trying until I said I did not want to hear any more about it.

I then arranged my own lawyer to help me deal with the aggression and lies which were going to take me away from my work for Alex and drain my emotional energy if I kept countering. They could have verified facts about what was there when I took the lease from the Agent's photographs. Nonetheless they accused me of causing screw holes in the window frames and replacing the blinds with curtains without permission. They seemed to want to try anything, so I explained in writing through my lawyer:

> The screw holes in the window frames are not caused by me. I did not remove any blinds from the two front bedrooms and the curtains were already installed as per the condition report photographs. It would seem that these screw holes were made when the windows had roman blinds. These blinds were removed from the front bedroom at some stage prior to my lease. Other windows

(family room and TV room) still had roman blinds when I took the lease. The agent independently arranged for these to be removed and for Holland blinds (cream coloured) to be installed as replacements. He installed the same kind of blinds in the two front rooms behind the curtains. I pointed out the screw holes now visible on the upper part of the window frames in the family and TV rooms but he said to not worry about them. The same kind of holes in the front two bedrooms would therefore be assumed to arise from old removed roman blinds.

I did not replace any blinds with curtains. I put new curtains on the existing curtain rails in the front two rooms when I noticed one of the curtains in the main bedroom was torn after the incident on 3 September. The only blind I installed is the one over the glass sliding door to the kitchen which I was happy to replace when Alex broke the winding cord to the old one (which was grey and old and not matching the blinds in the remainder of the room).

I did keep a tabulation of all that I did – the final on 16 December on vacating the house as follow:

Item	Work	Status
Smashed windows main bedroom, smashed glass front door.	Re-glazed, glass pieces swept up.	Repairs complete
Light switch main bedroom	Plastering and painting together with new switch. An	Electrician replaced and certified light

	electrician will not certify an old switch. It is not that she found fault with the old one.	switch. Painting complete. Note slight vertical wave in plaster to the left of the switch.
Braced towel rail main bathroom	The rail and wood brace have been removed and plastering with repainting undertaken. The rail placed in the toilet was removed earlier.	Old towel rail has been re-fitted on filled and repainted wall.
Shower door main bathroom	Shower door and side glass were replaced after removal but the door was too loose at the hinge on inspection by owner in November.	Shower door fixed professionally. Adjustments needed were slight raising of lower hinge hole and firm fixation of upper rail in left hand connection to vertical piece (pop rivet and silicon). No top capping is associated with this design of shower (see

		ensuite shower of same design).
Cupboard doors damaged	In the back bedroom, the cupboard doors were replaced on the right hand side and mended on the left. The pantry cupboard door closest to the front of the house was not damaged by me or Alex but had a gouge mark already there, which I sought to rectify while the other damaged door at the further end was replaced and painted.	Door work complete. Dent in RHS door to the pantry present at commencement of lease has been filled. Painting complete.
Bedroom doors damaged	The doors to the main bedroom and bedroom three were dented, noting there was an existing dent in the main bedroom door	Repairing and painting complete
Walls with hole damage	The plastering and painting along the main hall and back hall walls and in the back bedroom.	Work complete. Note with light coming in a certain direction, different paint textures can be observed,

		otherwise damage has been rectified.
Walls where scratched and scuffed or dirty	Some cleaning, spot plastering and patch painting done	Work complete. Note the back wall to the walk-in wardrobe is as presented in the condition report.
Carpet main bedroom	Spots of discolouration, assumed to be from capsicum spray, add to the discolouration of the high traffic areas of the carpet. Cleaning does not change the bleaching effect of the spray.	As no approval has been given for either the colour or the January installation, the quote obtained from Flooring company for new carpet in the Main bedroom is not acted on.
Main toilet	Damage to the fly screen was discovered during lease but before my son came. I presume someone tried to break in to achieve the bend in the frame.	A new frame and screen have been installed. The old toilet seat and cover were replaced.

I also told them that I had done some extra work:

- ceiling globes in the kitchen replaced
- the loose palings and slipped fence plinth on the east boundary repaired
- Additional stucco plants put in the garden bed.
- The new kitchen tap and bathroom amenities remained, as the landlord had not asked for their removal, as did the earlier new LED light fittings in several rooms fitted (compliance obtained) remain.
- a blind on the kitchen glass sliding door and new curtains on the existing rails in the main bedroom and bedroom 2 installed
- The front door given a coat of varnish on the outside. The glass panels replaced with translucent glass at the landlord's request after original glass was smashed
- The side gate fixed where it broke at the lower hinge due to lack of a stop to prevent the gate over-swinging
- The spots (unknown origin) on the south-east corner of the family room ceiling cleaned off.

I also admitted that a small mark existed where there was none evident in the condition report on a hall door, with its cause unknown and only belatedly noted as it was hidden while the door was in the cavity.

I did not receive the courtesy of a response from the landlord. I did not get my bond back. He did not give me receipts for the rent sent once he was managing the lease himself. I do not have any formal finalisation of the fiasco. I owe a lot to my brother for helping, at great inconvenience, for additional work to make sure the repairs were to a high standard.

I have told this story about the landlord to not only explain further why Alex could not return to Small Town, to either the rental house or his SDA, but also to give readers an idea of the extended ramifications of failures in the mental health system.

In the meantime, Alex had moved to very temporary accommodation in Northern Melbourne and had the benefits of his new antipsychotic medication. Alex was very keen to shop and go for walks. With an effort, on understanding Alex's improved capacities for being in the public, we were able to allow him walks in a park at Northern Melbourne. There was a wonderful area within walking distance of his accommodation with trees and bush as well as a basketball ring and other amenities.

It was such a pleasure for Alex, we used an outing to this park the day we had to move him again, this time to Western Melbourne in November, to reduce possible stress with the move. We packed his things while he was at the park. He came back in such a good mood he was quite calm when he was told about the move that day, to yet another place which was not his permanent home and where he might feel strange.

On having to vacate Northern Melbourne, we had run out of time to find somewhere appropriate for Alex to go. Ideally, we would not have accepted the Western Melbourne respite facility. The alternative of him living on the street was terrifying.

Chapter 14 Inexorable decline

November 2022 - February 2023

Alex coped with his move from Northern Melbourne to Western Melbourne very well but things were far from satisfactory. The facility had design faults and was not ready for someone moving in. The organisation running it seemed to be inexperienced and with poor business practices. The area was a disappointment with no parks within walking distance. There was no immediate uptake of Alex as a client in the local mental health clinic, possibly because again of a poor handover. When the psychiatric registrar did come to visit him at home, they displayed no background understanding of Alex. It was also while at Western Melbourne that Alex began reporting a new physical problem: "blank outs" he called them.

On reflecting about Alex since he left the Regional Hospital, and that he had been given cariprazine, I reported to the team on 1 December 2022:

Alex is so much better overall:

- more able to handle frustrations and disappointments
- more logical

- better meds compliance
- less volatile/angry
- speaking more politely
- next to no manic symptoms relating to delusions and rapid changes of emotion,
- sleeping better overall – only one night recently of taking to writing all night instead of getting to bed
- ready to apologise for bad behaviour.

Some other points made by others were:

- Increased capacity to follow directions / instructions. Serena gave the example where he was able to follow multiple steps, one by one, on how to solve a problem on his phone
- Able to engage in more complex tasks e.g. card making, cooking, arts and crafts, and shopping
- Increased tolerance for staff with dark coloured skin. He made a good connection with a Nigerian worker
- Alex is waking up most nights between 1-4 times, most commonly seeking staff reassurance or to use the toilet
- Intensity of behaviours of concern have significantly reduced – no staff injuries, seclusion not currently being used, no property damage.

This was great but Alex was not consistent. He could still be difficult to manage at times. He could be irritable because he hated being away from home with me, hated a loss of independence (as he remembered it) and hated not being in ACT. Despite the good signs, with the background of his physical problems and his lack of understanding what has happened over the last five years to change his life, I made the following qualifications to the good news:

- Alex's sleep is a problem and we are exploring sleep apnoea with GP but it is also related to multiple wakes due to urinary frequency (on diuretic on top of historic frequency) resulting in drowsiness during the day and irritability
- There has been no review of medicine overall since his arrival in Victoria, only additions to the list – is he over sedated for what he needs for symptoms?
- The trigger from young people being near is persisting. He believes that he is being called names (spastic and retard) even when such children/youths have not said anything at all nor perhaps even looked his way. It does not seem as if he is hallucinating in that he seems otherwise quite present in the moment. We have not resolved whether he is remembering a past event and re-experiencing the emotion?
- Because of unpredictability we continue to be concerned about taking him to public areas. When thinking he is being called names he reacts to them aggressively.
- We continue to be concerned about taking him shopping (besides mania he has always been afraid of running out, so shops excessively). Alex never does things in moderation.
- He has worsening leg pain
- He experiences some seizures regardless of valproate and clonazepam

- He shows poor compliance some days because he blames his tablets for feeling dopey, but has better compliance overall
- He exhibits extra salivation during the day.

Again, a poor handover

During November to December 2022, we again found that communication between mental health units was abysmal, meaning that we were not getting the timely help badly needed. There was an unforgiveable delay in getting mental health care for Alex, even though I had managed to get him to a GP in Western Melbourne who seemed thorough. Unfortunately, he was not in a position to immediately work through the long list: leg veins, cataract, neurologist for blank outs and valproate, sleep apnoea, podiatry. It was all a slow trawl; we got appointments but did not achieve specialist care before his death.

I received a call on 15 November from the area Mental Health Triage letting me know that Alex's transfer was on their radar. The lady gave me numbers for contact. This sounded promising compared to the move to Northern Melbourne, but I never knew what the real purpose of this call was, because subsequently nothing seemed to be happening. The numbers I tried to call sent me in circles and no one knew about Alex and the urgency.

It took until December for the mental health clinic in Western Melbourne to acknowledge Alex as their patient and visit him at home. A psychiatrist, Dr Q, and a case manager nurse came. I was present, as was the House Leader, Serena. It was a most unsatisfactory visit. I stated that Alex needed a review of his medication urgently: they needed to consider reducing the clozapine and increasing the cariprazine. Dr Q looked at me blankly and went on to fuss about Alex's trousers and shoes in front of him.

This was appalling: their job was medication, my job was clothing, and time was of the essence for his health. If she thought his clothing was so important and had only bothered to ask me, I could have explained, separately, that about Alex strict requirements either from quirks (such as wanting cargo pant pockets) to size requirements (e.g. swollen long feet calling for me to buy footwear online from America). The case manager had no idea about how to speak with Alex. She tried giving him a lecture about the need for exercise and staying healthy! She had been told earlier that there might be some difficulties getting Alex out of the house (perhaps not spelt out enough because it was in front of him) but did not connect that information with the need to adjust one's messages to him. Later that day Alex got very cross and agitated with workers for not taking him out since the nurse said he had to.

Physical ill-health and medication side-effects

Alex's physical health continued to decline. His diet was bad: too much sugar and other carbohydrates. He was often too tired to go for a walk even if an opportunity arose. His pain in his legs required constant painkillers. His legs were swollen and he kept his shoes and socks on 24/7 with the risk of fungal infections again. He still refused to shower. I do not think he had washed much while at Dhulwa and continued to refuse to in the community. One of his issues was a fear of falling which persisted from December to February 2023. Exacerbating this fear was an emergence of a blacking out phenomenon which was separate from the petit mal episodes. Each blank/blackout was very brief but could occur several times in a few minutes once started.

We did not know whether he was experiencing a lot of side effects from all his medicines. Without resolution and clarity of all the problems associated with his mix of medicines, we could not get improvement in his physical health.

Alex had been prescribed suvorexant to try to improve his sleeping but no one was monitoring this usage where monitoring was advised if he was also taking, clozapine, carbamazepine and/or cariprazine.

Clonazepam had been prescribed by Dr O at the same time as he prescribed cariprazine. Dr O did tell me that the dose of cariprazine would, or should be titrated up. But as I have detailed, there was never any continuity in care after that day so I do not think anyone had looked at his clonazepam either, for to increase the dose or to check whether it was contributing to negative effects. The side effects commonly listed for clonazepam include:

- drowsiness.
- dizziness.
- unsteadiness.
- problems with coordination.
- difficulty thinking or remembering.
- increased saliva.
- muscle or joint pain.
- frequent urination.

That is a good match with what Alex was experiencing.

An ongoing community problem was not being able to keep his trousers up once he had both hands on his camera, a constant companion when he was out. Because of his huge stomach there was no place for his waistband to grip, even with a smaller size and even with a belt. I bought braces after one day in a park when, following his visit to the Western Melbourne Clinic GP, he took pictures and members of the public wanted to call the police on seeing this man with trousers around his ankles getting loud and obvious. Alex never wore the braces and did not get out much thereafter anyway.

Sadly, Alice had to move on within her organisation at this stage. Alex had grown fond of her and she was missed. She bore the brunt of the professional challenge on realising she had a mentally ill client with no medical help, the Small Town reaction and being the front line when her Support Worker Organisation was the subject of baseless criticisms all round.

Alex felt himself sliding

Alex was not always able to articulate his symptoms but he felt sick a lot over Christmas and the 2023 New Year. Christmas Day was a family event and a disaster as we gathered in a local park with a picnic but Alex could not get himself up and ready to join us, for several reasons, including sedation. The PRN sedation was an overkill from carers that day.

He kept dialling 000 himself from late 2022 such that the emergency service was tired of him. He told me he was afraid he was going to die and needed their help. When I visited which was fairly often at this stage, I did observe that he had developed a need for care with similar needs to those in aged care.

I kept telling Alex he was not about to die. Was I not giving him the credibility he deserved? I told him about all the doctors, specialists and the dentist we had made arrangements for him to see. Christmas was stalling some things, but he would be looked after. I assured him we were looking after him.

I visited Alex on Boxing Day. He was really difficult, got aggressive and I reacted badly, wanting him so desperately to control his behaviour. What sort of life could he possibly have? On 28 December I left a message on the Western Melbourne Clinic case manager's phone saying that we wanted a family meeting. At our team meeting on 5 January, we talked about the frustrations of getting care and wondered how we could escalate the situation. We decided to wait until after the family meeting held on 11 January. We also talked yet again about what SDA opportunities there might be in Victoria to meet Alex's criteria. We agreed to ask around for opinions on which areas had good mental health services.

Alex was reluctant to let me go as usual on my visits. "You are my Mum! I am your son. I should be able to live at your place".

Alex typed up his thoughts wanting to be heard by his community doctors as shown on the next page. His words as read posthumously are very sad and poignant.

Hi from your Patient Alex James Cameron is somehow really feeling hugely a bit Dizzy and is feeling that will feel that could Fall Over downwards down to the ground very hard and instantly be life out with being very hurt with Crushed sore Muscles and Bones that's say if i had taken my tabs that is and my meds, if taken . I as Alex James Cameron myself has felt that to not take them at all so that voids falling down if taken tabs, and look i really hate taking the tabs that you have me, So i say to Stop ordering them from such a Collectable place, any more, Because Your tabs Supply is very not very good to me, and is getting to much that i do not Like also that myself feels that i feel the feeling to fall over to the ground, because of this taking of these tabs, and because it is that we only live once in real life, in life, and I'm to say that the tabs have me feeling very Dopafied or the feeling of being dopey for the few hours, of about it, and i really hate the way that these tabs get me into, and i should be ending up really doing other things besides just dopeing of in on bed every day like it feels me have, because it's like for the love of God, oh what have i been doing all this time, and gees i should have been doing my very heaps of Art and Craft all this time and not been doing unthoughtful things instead of bugering up my sparetime with the taking of my tabs and not doing thoughtful interesting things for Friends and Family, instead of just sitting on my bed, because my very famous nice mum really needs me Son Alex James Cameron to really get my acts up to be the best son of all times, and be the one to be very Special, and not very Shameful, and to get my Mum proud of me and not be very Shameful, and Disappointed or very Disappointing, and that the tabs are very really Dumb, to be very Stupid, that i really hate taking them

Last ditch effort

My daughter-in-law and Serena attended the meeting on 11 January with me. Together with the staff we had met or previously spoken to at Western Melbourne clinic, Dr R a consultant psychiatrist, attended. There was some initial discussion about the team assigned to Alex and contact information. We highlighted the over-sedation and possible narcolepsy. Dr R wanted to consider his thyroid hormone status which I acknowledged could be a concern if the way he was taking thyroxine precluded proper absorption, but I really thought they should be looking at his high clozapine used in conjunction with his anticonvulsants while we were trying to investigate his sleep apnoea. We talked about getting Alex to a neurologist and I explained I had left this because of the housing moves and it was difficult to get Alex to appointments without an incident. Valproate and clonazepam had been prescribed by the psychiatrists and not the neurologists anyway.

Nonetheless, with the help of my daughter-in-law, I immediately made a concerted effort to get expert neurology help for Alex. It did take a few tries to get an adequate referral from his GP and try to make sure Alex was seen as soon as possible.

I pointed out at the January meeting that he seemed to have a paradoxical reaction of agitation despite a medicines regime expected to have some sedative effect. Valproate, for example, was supposed to be a mood stabiliser. Dr R said autism cannot be treated with medicine! My daughter-in-law quickly came back with "But he is manic!" Thus, this notion that Alex's mania symptoms were not mental health symptoms had carried through to Western Melbourne Clinic. Dhulwa, then the Regional Health Service, then the Regional Hospital, then Northern Mental Health Unit had a lot to answer for. The perpetuation of this attitude seemed to arise from the habit of just reading what the previous doctor said instead of doing a renewed assessment and re-appraisal, and from not listening to the person who knew Alex best. There was a kind of group think occurring, with the group being the mental health clinical staff over several facilities. The Victorian Dual-disability Expert upheld the need for a different approach in pointing out to me the error in their diagnosis.

Was anyone noticing?

When Alex started complaining about being "super cold" all the time, even though it was summer I was worried. That is what he complained of for weeks leading up to his NMS in January 2022. No one had been able to say this temperature perception was linked to NMS but I thought it worth the Western Melbourne house having a thermometer to be able to monitor Alex's temperature from then on.

It was only in January that Western Melbourne Clinic measured Alex's actual blood level of clozapine and found it above therapeutic level. Dr R from Western Melbourne Clinic dropped Alex's clozapine dosage from 750 mg to 700 mg per day (still high) and did not increase cariprazine which she said she might do the following month. She wanted to do things slowly. In hindsight we know we did not have time for her belated start to her ideal schedule.

Alex had been prescribed high doses of clozapine and valproate on discharge from Dhulwa and no one in Victoria had checked the reasons for these doses or the risks involved. My guess is that valproate was regarded as a useful medicine for Alex, being both a mood stabiliser and an anticonvulsant, and Dhulwa kept the clozapine level high to aim at a therapeutic level while the valproate increased clozapine metabolism. No questions asked in Victoria. No one mentioned anything about the potential role of valproate in NMS.

One problem with prescribing valproate was Alex's compliance. In July to August Alex frequently threw out his valproate. All along, Alex stated that he did not like the purple tabs (or the red liquid) even when compliant with other medication. We have no map of whether the variable compliance did affect, or what kind of effects this had on, his behaviours or physical health. Once he was better after being given cariprazine, his compliance with valproate improved, but then worsened with his physical decline and distress at being in the Respite house. Maybe taking more valproate was really a bad idea. Alex reacted against it anyway. By January Alex was going for longer periods without valproate. There was a two week period in January 2023 when Alex refused to take valproate and during that time, he was better mentally than he had been for a long time. When the GP ordered a blood level of valproate, he found it zero at this time of course. Alex said that it made him feel funny so he did not want to take it.

With lower valproate, his clozapine was not as rapidly metabolised and would be at higher levels. Higher levels likely increased the risk of Alex contracting NMS again. NMS is not a dose-dependent phenomenon, but higher doses are a risk factor[11].

Doubtful certification as respite SDA

Alex was not living in a good respite facility conducive to best care in Western Melbourne. During Alex's stay there, the required communication between the Support Worker Organisation and the respite facility was fraught. It was also strained between the facility and the Support Coordinator. There were several attempts by Serena to negotiate smoothly over difficulties with the house, but the facility organisation showed little willingness to behave in a professional manner. Staff there were not willing in many ways.

We thought the facility created barriers to appropriate disability care include the following:

1. Not built to robust standards as advertised
    - Door hinges easily became dislodged: bedroom and bathroom doors became hazards
    - Staff egress restriction with the external door design
    - Fixtures easily came off walls: shelf in bathroom fell on floor, intercom unit placed next to toilet was easily knocked with normal toilet use (neither ever fixed)
    - Glass in living room was not reinforced
    - Lightweight furniture
    - Easily knocked porcelain pot plant on bedroom floor

---

[11] Reference: Caroff SN, Mann SC. Neuroleptic malignant syndrome. Med Clin North Am 1993; 77:185.

- Bed had easily removable metal mattress-holding bars as potential weapons and if even one was removed for safety the mattress was impossible to keep on the bed
- Easily removable sliding cupboard doors (taken out in original modifications though)
- Poor design in bathroom with small basin and no bench for articles behind door when open
- Inability to make staff area secure in original design and had to be reinforced under arrangements by Support Organisation
- Door to exit the client's bedroom into the courtyard was flimsy and did not close properly
- Wall pictures had to be removed
- Wheelchair-friendly adjustable bench section in kitchen but no other design accommodating wheelchair bound clients: e.g. rungs in wardrobe high and only steps at front with alternative exit only through garage

2. Basic domicile deficiencies
    - Ongoing short circuiting of appliances in kitchen
    - No key for accessing mail in the letterbox
    - Lengthy time to get hot water in client area
    - No bedside units for radio, water bottle etc. (no communication on what furniture client should provide either)
    - Poorly installed washing machine with moving bolts not removed, so that it jumped around into the hallway and made a shocking noise
    - No internet for months even though promised and eventually only partial service with addition of a WIFI extender

- Laundry was inaccessible for three weeks, ostensibly because respite facility needed someone to remove other client possessions from that cupboard.

3. Health and safety issues
   - No outlook/claustrophobic gaol feel – depressing environment for someone with limited mobility
   - Extraordinary smell from toilet at times
   - No walking space unless in open street (patches outside called courtyards of little use)
   - Slip hazard with fake grass in said courtyard
   - No handrail on front steps and other difficulties for someone with a walking frame
   - Inability to open windows for fresh air – no access to open windows is technically considered as a restrictive practice.

4. Failures to correct issues
   - Several requests had to be made for anything needing to be fixed.
   - Bathroom door hinges broken for 2 plus months
   - Garage door did not close correctly for weeks upon coming to the unit and then the 2nd unit had the same issue.
   - The badly installed washing machine noise had to be tolerated for weeks
   - Maintenance slow to be undertaken
   - No keys: windows an ongoing issue and for front door.
   - Support Organisation had to get its own keys cut for the sliding door @ $200 vs the ridiculous quote given by the respite facility
   - Internet failure never fully corrected and only some usage with extra work by the Support Organisation.

5. Difficulties over requirement to move units within the complex
   o Change of moving dates causes massive confusion including with back and forth changes
   o Only with repeated explanations from the Support Worker Organisation were modifications to the new property commenced and completed.
   o Locks not suitable in second unit
   o Organisation put the reinforcement latch on the outside of Alex's bedroom (we would be locking Alex's into his room!) instead of inside the staff room. They failed to take proper note of the request or to anticipate that locking Alex up would not be good Support Worker practice.

6. Communication poor
   o Never available to answer calls, SMS, emails and seemed to prefer phone over email as there was no record of their sometimes, offensive language.
   o Respite organisation management did not communicate when trades or their staff were going to enter property (often found maintenance handy girl smoking in garage if we had garage door open to let staff in).
   o when making requests for the internet to be fixed the Support Worker organisation house coordinator was advised to be solution focused, not mention past issues and to move forward

7. Unprofessional behaviour
   o Shopping orders became an issue when constant pleading with management to pay for orders as part of initial agreement were ignored

- Support Organisation had to organise own fixing of sliding door locks with repeated failure of respite facility to respond
- Failure to understand instructions for invoicing: Invoicing sent to NDIA planner, despite directions otherwise
- Poor language in email to NDIA under wrongful notion they the respite organisation had been aggrieved:
- emails to plan manager threatening legal action for 'late payment', which was misrepresenting what happened
- Repeatedly late for meeting appointments
- No understanding of the role of communication in working together

8. Poor understanding of disability sector
   - No sensitivity to client needs and risks with the forced move: thought he could move without notice
   - Support Organisation told to move him when he is out and he will not know the difference
   - Requested Alex to pay for frosting to the windows after securing NDIA payments for SIL staff they were not providing

On 12 January 2023 we were told by the respite facility that Alex would have to move to another of their units among the four units in a row. Consistent with the poor capabilities they had already exhibited, the facility management showed hopelessness in the following weeks trying to plan and organise this move. First, we had to work through any issues that might need modification prior to Alex moving in. The availability of the new unit kept changing, assessment opportunities kept changing, the ability to inspect reported modification and the move date kept changing. Alex was in ICU Western Melbourne Hospital when the move was actually made and he personally never went there.

Maintaining care not easy as Alex felt worse

The team managed to get Alex to visit a vascular surgeon on 13 January. That doctor said he should wear compression socks, elevate his legs at night and have physiotherapy – all the things we had tried previously. If Alex refused or was resistant because of all his other issues, we were not going to get improvement in his swollen legs. We also managed to get Alex to the sleep study clinic but he was not able to tolerate the placement of the leads for a home study. As a follow up we investigated options such as a hospital stay study. Alex had repeated incidents of conjunctivitis for which I repeatedly got chloramphenicol drops. Effectively administering these for treatment was almost impossible. Alex was not easy.

Alex pleaded for a permanent home. He felt as if all the promises for him to have his very own place had been a sham. His third temporary home! He saw himself in a situation far from his dreams. He felt as if he did not deserve it. He thought he was a good person who only wanted to do good, creative and useful things. This is not what should happen in people's lives! "It was not supposed to be this way Mum!"

To be still in a temporary home, one which locked him inside so much, was distressing for him. He seemed to lose the drive to even go for a walk sometimes, so I wanted to encourage every opportunity. One Saturday in January while I was visiting, I was trying to execute a plan to have a short walk. I had talked about it the previous day with Alex and Serena.

Alex was really slow to get ready and it approached time for the change of shift. The day shift told me about how they were trying to stimulate Alex to get going. But their method was to urge him to walk from his bedroom to the kitchen as a condition to be met for an external walk. I was appalled. It was not up to them to equate the two. It would not be the same motivation! Then with Alex ready to go they said it was too close to their shift finishing.

When the new shift arrived, I said we were going for a walk. I had pushback from one worker. He said he knew nothing about that so I told him the house leader Serena had agreed. He should have had a handover from the day shift. He went away and came back accepting the plan. He was not constructive in making it happen. He did not want to help Alex get down the front steps as it seemed he had some aversion to touching him, so I asked him to take the walker while I helped Alex, and the other worker managed the door. We had not gone two steps on the footpath before the reluctant worker asked Alex if he wanted to go back.

I kept it going and Alex had a good walk, even if slow. When he saw some people on the path outside their house, he volunteered to walk to the other side of the road because he said he did not want to disturb them. He kept wanting to turn into another street while his reluctant carer tried to dissuade him. I wanted Alex to walk as far as possible. However, when Alex indicated he wanted to head to the shops I suggested he had better go home now. I knew the carers were nervous about Alex in shops. This staff reaction occurred now regardless of whether he showed any signs of mania on the day. I had further disagreement with that worker when we returned, but the main problem was his failure to see the importance for Alex's health of taking a walk. I said he should be walking every day.

I had further evidence that some of the support workers had been too negative or did not behave appropriately so that Alex would get out of his prison. The staff on duty the next morning would not give Alex his breakfast and then would not give him his painkiller medicine unless he walked to the kitchen. Serena had to go to the house (Sunday) to sort it out. It seemed to me that while most of the staff had started well with Alex, they had grown too wary while not taking appropriate notice of his mental health state and symptoms to respond accordingly. I do not think they understood mania: only agitation versus calm.

Dr R visited on 21 January and took time to listen to Alex and consider matters such as his legs. This psychiatrist proposed that Alex halve his dose of valproate for which she wrote the prescription, not waiting for any neurologist. And she asked Alex about taking it in tablet form which he agreed to. We did not have to obtain any more tablets from the pharmacy as there are quite a few still in store from the time we switched to liquid form. She talked about reducing clozapine and increasing cariprazine. This was very hopeful.

First visit to Western Melbourne hospital

A side effect of clozapine is constipation. Alex was taken to Emergency at Western Melbourne Mercy Hospital who diagnosed a bowel blockage and kept him overnight on 26 January. We aggressively treated this so that his blockage was rectified. Of significance, given his pneumonia in February was the identification among the investigations made on that visit to ED was scarring on the lungs. The GP, a January relief doctor, to whom I spoke about this did not think it was much to worry about.

The support workers had started so well in Small Town under extremely trying circumstances and now they were jaded. I was finding more things they did less than adequate. I only found out about the discharge when Alex rang me. The night shift had not reported what was happening and they did not bring all Alex's clothing back with him. You can imagine the upset with someone always worried about his things! Alex yelled at me, but one of the good workers later calmed him down. The hospital kept looking for the clothing thanks to this worker chasing it up.

The hospital was originally remiss in demanding he remove clothing for an ECG, causing dramatic scenes that night. They did not do the ECG anyway. The hospital then did not make sure staff had the clothing in a bag in their hands or at least under their watchful eye. The clothing was lost. I complained that staff were not keeping track when they should know Alex's phobias about people taking his stuff!

A good sign of the helpfulness of the Western Melbourne Hospital was a call I received at the end of January from a social worker there who asked for more information about Alex. She asked for anything that could help them communicate with Alex and asked if she could have some advice about his conditions on record. This was quite a contrast to the earlier Regional Hospital.

Disability staff needed help when nurses really required

One night, before we realised Alex did need urgent medical attention, staff were not focussed on really reading his symptoms. When I spoke to a worker, he said Alex is always complaining of these symptoms as if inured to his complaints. I also had occasion to find night staff not answering the staff phone after Alex rang me to say he could not get a response when calling for their help early that morning.

One or two new staff who had good potential were being recruited. A new training session was introduced. Serena and I discussed what else might be required regarding improving support staff at this stage. We did not lose momentum in seeking the best for Alex.

A lot of work also went into planning the theatre trip which was very exciting. We had a team meeting with the case manager at Western Melbourne on 2 February. We were given an update on Alex's medication. We had some discussion about the Behaviour Support Plan and staff awareness given some comments made by hospital staff. Serena commented about some new staff joining the crew. I was told that my method of seeking mental health help via email was not the normal method! It was advised that Alex should have weight scales for observation of possible fluid fluctuations. The issue of the pending review of Alex's NDIS Plan was also raised. We were still looking for an SDA! All these matters became redundant concerns.

After the explanation above about the lack of outings for Alex, it should be obvious that getting Alex to see Mary Poppins at the theatre in the middle of the City Melbourne on 8 February was a special joy. He took his walker for confidence in getting about but he was in great form. He behaved so well and enjoyed the day that we thought he would be able to get out much more! I gave him a big hug before I left him in that good spot at the theatre to fly to Hobart as Ewen and my daughter-in-law were sick and needed help with my young grandson.

Chapter 15 The end result
February - March 2023

Three days after the trip to see Mary Poppins, Alex started vomiting frequently and at volume, and by early Sunday 12 February he was clearly ill. I was still in Hobart so Serena came to the house to handle the urgent need for medical assistance. Alex told me by phone "I am very ill Mum". I agreed and my stomach lurched but I was not panicking. That was Day 1.

On the same day, in between my calls about Alex I also had calls from Canberra because my ex-husband had fallen requiring stitches in his lip. His new wife needed me to speak to the ambulance officer and then to the doctor at the Emergency Department because of her language problems. I had one phone call after another for most of the day. Keeping in contact with me, Serena arranged for a telehealth appointment for Alex which confirmed the need for an ambulance. The ambulance services did not want to attend, having previously thought that Alex was malingering, and, when they did attend, Serena had to insist that they take Alex to the Emergency Department. They eventually acknowledged that, given his constipation, vomiting and temperature, they really should take him.

I would come to regret not bringing my return flight to Melbourne forward from Monday to Sunday.

The diagnosis, like the earlier trip to the Western Melbourne Hospital, was about his bowel. Despite the intensive treatment with fibre and bowel wall stimulants, and apparent success in relieving constipation over the previous two weeks, a blockage was seen as the problem. After a CT scan apparently showed a catch in his bowel, the decision was to undertake keyhole surgery to release this. The communication to me from the doctor was that this sort of catch of an unusual looping in the bowel was often from a congenital condition that does not always manifest with a blockage, but now it had. The surgery was scheduled for Monday morning. I would arrive in Melbourne to visit him by late Monday afternoon on Day 2.

The doctor was at pains to say that the blockage was not a clozapine-induced constipation. This was important in terms of our guilt that the recent response to constipation was, possibly, inadequate or carelessly monitored.

There were many things to confront at this stage in Alex's life. Not the least was his inability to communicate, but there were signs he was not oblivious to the threat on his life. The overarching theme for me was the double thinking required on whether there was an inevitable path downhill for his illness and whether it was Alex's frailties or doctors' biased views taking charge. I felt there was bias because of their emphasis on the condition he was in immediately prior to this ICU admission, which set a low bar for what kind of recovery was a possible target. I could not know what Alex was going through and whether he really had any fight left, although there were hints that he knew of his perilous situation. By the time sedation was able to be reduced for him to react visibly, I knew he was suffering and hope was disappearing. The staff reports and comments were a string of parallel positive and negative.

We had thought everything was positive prior to 12 February. We had reached a point of such comparative success, such joy at the successful trip to the theatre, that we were completely unprepared for what happened next. Despite the January trip to the Western Melbourne Hospital for severe constipation and the calls made by Alex himself to triple zero fearing serious illness since November, his reduced mobility and waning interest in his usual pursuits such as photography, we had not perceived a life-threatening physical state for Alex.

He had said a few times to me that he was afraid of dying whilst in Western Melbourne to which I had responded, "You are not going to die from these difficulties". I assured Alex that we were following up his various complaints with the GP and specialists. I had said I was sorry there were delays but we would get treatment. I was particularly sorry that we had a delay in getting neurology help because I agreed with Alex that the valproate side-effects were a problem, and we certainly needed to understand what these new 'blank-outs' were and their connection to his absence seizures.

This is the Intensive Care Unit!

I was warned by a few staff on arriving at the hospital on 13 February (Day 3) that seeing Alex at this stage might be confronting. I had experienced visiting Alex and other seriously ill people in hospital multiple times and had certainly experienced extensive caring for Alex whilst in the Canberra ICU previously. Nonetheless, I slowly took in the challenge of this kind of hospital care with intubation attached to breathing machine, nasogastric tube, urinary catheter, and venous and arterial lines in place. Alex was sedated and did not respond to my presence.

There seemed to be good news in the subsequent report that there was no bowel blockage to be found once they had opened him up. The doctor told me that they would probably remove the tube to his lungs the following morning. This would mean removal of sedation so that he would pick up the breathing on his own. The doctor asked that I could be there at the time of Alex's arousal in case he was scared and upset.

There were several doctors giving me reports – most were consultant ICU experts but some were registrars. It was hard to keep track of the role and status of any doctor in contact at a given time. Different doctors held the position of 'team leader doctor' for Alex and I tried to establish relationships with each. I did not keep a diary but some exchanges with particular doctors were embedded in my memory. Surely this physical health setback would all be over soon I told myself, so I would not need notes and would get back to the long-term complex, demanding task of improving his mental health with minimal side effects. Perhaps it just seemed like the multiple previous hospital stays to me.

The ensuing six weeks were filled with watching and waiting and trying to follow the balancing act the doctors were undertaking between sedating, and removing sedation. They were trying to achieve the best conditions for allowing Alex to breathe on his own, while not getting so disinhibited that it would be counterproductive to recovery and rehabilitation. I was never really sure whether they were in a position, having not known him prior to this admission, to assess what level of agitation he might display. They had experienced his awakening sufficiently in the first week to observe him trying to pull lines and tubes and kick the end of his bed.

Concurrent with this underlying juggle was the shifting in awareness of symptoms and consequently of diagnoses. On Day 3 the morning after surgery, Alex was diagnosed with aspiration pneumonia, thought at that stage to be due to breathing in vomitus at the time of intubation. Identification of the causative bacteria revealing two antibiotic resistant bacteria by Day 7. More suitable antibiotics were able to be prescribed once sensitivity tests could be performed.

Extubation was planned for Day 4. I was there as requested but then was told to wait. The respiratory doctor then thought Alex was not ready. On Day 5 a bronchoscopy was performed. A shift to the prone position was tried as apparently this had proved a successful treatment for those suffering from COVID-19. On Day 6 the outlook was brighter. But Days 8-11 proceeded without any removal or little removal of sedation. I kept coming and trying to make sure Alex knew I was there even while he could not indicate he knew. No extubation. I was kept strictly to visiting hours for spending time with Alex.

Someone rang me from the hospital one morning asking about Alex's previous admission to ICU. I explained it was in Canberra Hospital for Neuroleptic Malignant Syndrome (NMS). The caller said they would get the notes from Canberra Hospital, explaining they just wanted to cover the possibility they had missed something. My antennae for further twists in the story were raised.

Dr S was friendly and knew the importance of communication to the patient's family, but he gave the slight impression he was withholding something all the time. I was anxious and suspicious. Dr S chatted about the various symptoms and Alex's inability to drop his temperature despite being treated with antibiotics. As frequently as they could, they were checking for signs of remaining or new infections. ICU was a place for acquired infections. I mentioned Alex had had NMS just over twelve months prior to this in which his temperature was raised. Dr S asked me what NMS was.

Not again!

On Day 11 I was asked suddenly to come to a family meeting the following day (Day 12) at 2 pm with a new lead doctor, Dr T. I was eventually ushered into a small lounge accompanied by Nurse Experience whom I had not met previously, and Dr S. I dialled Serena to be on speaker phone. Dr T was about to make a statement of Alex's situation when he asked me instead to summarise. He accepted my summary of Alex's shifting diagnosis and persistent symptoms and continued. He said we could add the measurement of high levels of creatine kinase linked to muscle breakdown to the list of symptoms, leading them to diagnose a new bout of NMS. This was made despite Alex not having the muscle rigidity usually associated with NMS. It is not that there is a definitive diagnostic profile for NMS but with the high CK level it was the best possible explanation. His body was burning up again. Devastation.

Dr T said "Have you heard of it?" I looked at him. He repeated the question. I echoed, "Have I heard of it – I was the one who mentioned it to Dr S here. NMS is what Alex had last year." I thought *where does this man think I was while Alex contracted NMS and was in ICU last year? Does he think I just came into Alex's life for this latest illness? Does he think I would not have known what Alex had last year?* I said I was taken aback because I really thought Alex would be much safer from NMS without the lithium that he had been on for the last occasion, given the way he had been on clozapine (without lithium) for twenty years without contracting NMS. And the hospital's doctors had been apparently, clearly, identifying non-NMS symptoms until now.

I held my head with my hands and Dr T reached for the tissue box. I told him I was not going to cry. The anguish I felt was numbing with the full understanding of the setback this was. I said I understood they would have to remove his antipsychotics and this did not bode well for physical recovery either. He said he had already stopped his antipsychotics. We talked a bit about what symptoms might emerge and what capacity they had to manage him and the potential need for an admission to a suitable mental health facility in a few weeks. I was thinking of the road being doubly hard yet again but not of there being no road forward. Permanent institutionalisation was my big fear at that stage. I really did not fully appreciate yet the repercussions of the renewed physical challenge!

Dr T then went to the subject of end-of-life planning and asked me about the value in fighting for Alex's survival. How hard should they try? I gave a speech. I set my position as guardian which meant spokesperson for Alex's wishes. I detailed his desire to live, his desires to do so many things, his interests in life and the great spirit and determination he had shown to live in the community again after being incarcerated in mental health facilities since 2017. I said Alex should not be discriminated against because of his disabilities, that we had been working on those disabilities and he needed still to be given the chance to recover to continue that process. I did not go into detail about how so much had been taken from him in the name of health, that it was unfair to then say he should have a limited opportunity for best treatment as a consequence of those health failures to care for him. Perhaps I should have. I asked Serena to provide her comments on Alex. She took the opportunity to reiterate my assessment and talk about there being so much that Alex should be valued for.

On the way out, Nurse Experience spoke close to me thanking me for my words, saying the doctors needed to hear that. I wondered what alternative scenario they had built up before my words.

I was very happy when Dr T was not on duty, especially because it was mostly then that Dr U was lead consultant for Alex. Dr V also drew confidence. He agreed with me that Alex's life was worth fighting for.

On Day 13 Serena visited Alex while I took a break to help with a working bee in Melbourne as part of my son, Ewen's, permanent move to Hobart. Serena noted Alex was aware enough to squeeze her hand. His eyes watered and Alex did not usually cry much. I received a call that he had developed pressure sores on his ears. Pressure sores were a constant risk against which they went to a lot of trouble to keep moving him. Day 14 Alex was said to be breathing better requiring less oxygen. Alex opened his eyes on Day 15. By Day 16 there was still no decision to extubate. His temperature showed improvement then increased again.

Serena and I packed up Alex's belongings from his temporary accommodation realising we would have to cancel the lease. We were weeks away from Alex needing discharge to living in the community. I was informed of the decision to switch from the tube to a tracheostomy on Day 18 (Dr V).

Hospital straining to find answers

Serena's internet search on NMS revealed that valproate does not have a passive role and could even be a contributor to NMS. I relayed this to a young doctor and again to Dr V the next day who was very puzzled about Alex not showing a drop in temperature, despite nearly a week off antipsychotics. Dr V agreed it would be worth removing valproate since under the current circumstances, absence seizures were a low priority. The persistent raised temperature was a conundrum.

At this stage, the hospital communicated that a decision had been made to allow support workers, who would be familiar faces to Alex, to visit him in the ICU. Given that there was now huge uncertainty about Alex's mood and degree of agitation when off sedation, or even with sedation but off antipsychotics, we were worried about the ability of those who had known him medicated to deal with him and help keep him calm.

Also on Day 18 I tried connecting the ICU medical team to the neurologist at the Alfred, whom we had recently introduced to Alex's complex issues with seizures, behaviour issues and mania. I was never told whether the contact was actually achieved. Nonetheless ICU staff certainly needed guidance on how to proceed regarding adequate, but not too much, sedation.

On Day 19, ICU introduced a body cooling system with wrap around water cooled compartments. They reported that they tried reducing the sedation again but Alex got distressed. I was not present to witness what form this took. I do not know whether allowing some level of distress but still achieving other aims was possible. Alex's normal state was anxiety. They operated on the basis that Alex's exhibitions of distress were too counterproductive. Sedation was increased again. Alex's weakened breathing system was explained to me. Efforts to get him to breathe on his own were becoming more difficult. I did not quite understand at this stage that recovery from having to rely on the tracheostomy was looking more and more difficult. People who do not have Alex's complications can find it difficult to overcome the tracheostomy. Nonetheless I was being told positive anecdotes about people making a full recovery including learning to speak again.

On Day 22 the report was that Alex's temperature was down and oxygen regulation was better. I was thinking I needed to tell Dr V that two data points do not make a trend but I wanted to hear the positive.

Days 23 – 26: The need to explore sedation for someone no longer on required antipsychotics, whilst facilitating recovery, was more explicit and urgent. I suggested that they contact Dr Victorian Dual-Disability Psychiatrist whom I had engaged late 2022 to advise on Alex's psychiatric treatment. This psychiatrist would be the best person for advice now because she had been extremely thorough in examining Alex's disability and psychiatric records back to childhood. The Victorian dual-disability psychiatrist was able to advise the hospital psychiatrist that an antidepressant to reduce anxiety was definitely not the answer. There were enough data on those similar to Alex with dual disability to warn of increases in mania with such an approach.

I obtained agreement for ICU doctors, the hospital psychiatrist, the community mental health unit that had picked up Alex's care from October 22 (on paper) to have a video conference with Dr Victorian Dual-disability Psychiatrist. This meeting was held on Day 28. Unfortunately, the technology left out the community mental health group which really needed to be party to the discussion if they had learnt anything about Alex and if they would resume care on discharge.

We covered Alex's developmental history which was consistent with autism, but not Intellectual Disability because of his childhood IQ of 109. Alex's apparent scores progressively declined over many years, his seizures increased, and his mental health deteriorated. It would seem that Alex's diagnosis was more accurately a neurodegenerative disease linked to his mutation. Intellectual Disability might have been a useful term to distinguish cognitive disability from physical disabilities, but it was not accurate medically, and meant that Alex's cognitive strengths and difficulties were not assessed. The label of Intellectual Disability is a trigger for diagnostic overshadowing in the health sector. I was still learning.

It was evident that this hospital too had continued in the mistaken belief that Alex's recent aggression was not due to being mentally ill. We had discussed in the video meeting the need for reduction of sedation while being fearful of emerging anxiety and aggression in such circumstances. Alex could not immediately, if ever, be resumed on antipsychotics because of the risk of NMS again. The hospital psychiatrist responded to the Victorian dual-disability psychiatrist's suggestion of Electroconvulsive Therapy (ECT) for the anticipated re-bound psychosis by saying "but his problem is *behaviours*". It is understood that ECT is not indicated for behaviours. He was denying that the target while sedation was being removed was mental illness. There was no reception to the dual disability expert's contribution.

The recommendation for ECT also covered its potential use in treating the NMS but the hospital did not take it further. One of the doctors later commented to me that Alex was not in a state to be taken to theatre for anaesthetisation in preparation for ECT or any other treatment. The pharmaceutical approach normally used for NMS was not effective for Alex, so treatment of whatever he had, proved impossible. His temperature stayed high.

Sedation was changed from fentanyl to propofol. It was all futile.

I had contact from ACT Health that week, as they wanted to arrange a meeting. In Melbourne if necessary. I told ACT Health that Alex was seriously ill and I would let them know if and when such a meeting was possible. I had missed the news, and did not know until I returned to the ACT, about the release by nurses of Alex's ACT hospital records, together with those of several patients, to WorkSafe and their union, and to private email addresses. There were more things afoot to haunt me it seemed.

Serena made a poster of photos of Alex to hang in his room. When a nurse had suggested this the previous week, I thought she was thinking it would help Alex, which was doubtful in my opinion, and could even stress him for the contrast to his current situation. She then explained it was for the staff! They needed to know that Alex was a person, a person with a life, family and friends and was recently mobile. He was not just an inert entity. Apparently it worked.

Alex had also given the impression with his unkempt appearance that he was completely uncared for at the time of his admission! The nurses thought his long-haired, unwashed, fungal infected state was because of lack of care. One nurse had even given Serena a lecture about it. Health people do not understand that if a client does not want to wash, a disability support worker cannot make him. And there is no way they would have understood why Alex would not be wanting to wash or would want to wear his shoes 24/7.

We continued with Alex awake more

Serena's visit on Day 28 allowed me to have another break. Alex had periods of being awake. Serena and I had both noticed unusual jerking movements at about this time, starting in his shoulders and moving to his abdomen. A nurse thought it might have been shivering. We were not convinced. Temperature was 39.6. Clozapine assays were only done on Tuesdays so we had to wait until after Day 31 for another check on whether the blood levels were indeed dropping or clozapine was still causing NMS. Infections were still on doctors' minds. Serena commented on the mixed messages we were getting with nursed generally optimistic while Dr S sounded more negative. This doctor's most positive message was, "there is a very long row to hoe".

I had asked Dr S whether Alex might have actually had NMS from his presentation in the Emergency Department. He said we could not know that! I understood we could not know that definitely but I considered it worth thinking through and developing theories. Why would Alex just develop NMS *AFTER* admission which had been about the apparent bowel problem and then pneumonia? In fact, vomiting and pneumonia go hand in hand with NMS. As a scientist I put forward hypotheses. Doctors are too guarded about grey areas because they think lay people just want, and can only deal with, black and white. If Alex had NMS, it was not following a common profile.

Days 28 to 30 comprised the March long-weekend for the Labour Day holiday in Melbourne. Dr U was off duty including for the Friday video conference, with Dr V as stand-in. No one was upbeat any more. The hospital arranged a visit to the ICU balcony as a change of scene for Alex. The facilities on the balcony allow for all the connections and oxygen required. He seemed to enjoy it and they tried it on another day but then he seemed totally opposed to going outside. His temperature was still high. Dr V definitely did not want Alex kept on sedation. Dr V had made a referral for Alex to go to the Alfred Hospital where they had a specialist ICU for such difficult cases struggling to get off a breathing machine. There was no bed there at that stage.

I had been trying various forms of communication with Alex such as asking questions to which he could respond yes or no with blinks or hand squeezes, which staff also tried. I tried progressing to asking him to point to things written on a clipboard. Nothing worked consistently. I could see him mouthing "mum" most times I entered his room. Sometimes his mouthing and noises was an indication of something distressing him. I failed in lip reading. We had some success with working out when and where he was in pain and whether we should ask the nurse for more pain killer. My encouragement to hold a pen to write his own message was a complete failure. I do not know whether this was a loss of will or whether the muscle fatigue had gone as far as his hand.

When he was in distress in this period, I found perhaps it was of most comfort to him if I cradled his whole head in my arms. He was crying frequently. The nurses had worked out for sensory comfort to keep a cloth wrap on his forehead. One or two nurses said Alex was always more settled when I visited.

Many nurses came and went with their long shifts. Some had several shifts with Alex. These ICU nurses were the most hard-working professional and thorough nurses I had witnessed – twelve-hour shifts and no toilet break unless they could get a temporary stand-in. There was always something to do for

Alex's care. It was relentless for the whole shift, and they were mostly in the room, but also with lots on notes to write at the console just outside his room.

When I saw nurses showing signs of distance when Alex was emerging from sedation, I explained, "He has feelings. He is crying which is not like him!".

I tried to tell Dr S at one stage that Alex had said in January that he was afraid of dying, as I wanted to indicate to them that he probably thought he was dying then, so that staff could appreciate his emotional state. Dr S said people die all the time and shrugged. He missed my point: I was not saying Alex thought he should never die. I was saying Alex felt something was seriously wrong with his health well before the admission. I should have said to him that Alex was afraid because he had premonitions he was going to die, of his conditions he himself felt to be life threatening.

The reality

A sudden downturn in hope occurred on Day 31. Dr U took me aside for a long talk through the issues. She had concluded there was no second round of infections for which they had been checking. His temperature was not coming down. He was not able to have reduced breathing support let alone independence from the machine. He did not have obvious psychotic symptoms under the degree of sedation. His diaphragm was weak. He was distressed every time they tried to get him to breathe on his own. He was prone to infections and progressively weaker the longer he was on the machine. Most people cared for in ICU, if they survive, are only kept there three days. We were in Alex's fifth week in the ICU.

Nonetheless, Dr U had explored external expert advice and would continue exploring and trying to find a solution.

When Dr U said they would keep trying, I naively had visions of weeks of Alex somehow held in the same state. How long was Dr U talking about when the pattern has been a holding-on in many ways? I wanted to know whether this meant he would not need me for short periods. I explained I had personal matters to attend to after the unexpected long period away from my home such as a need for a dentist and Serena would stand in for me for a rush trip back to Canberra. Dr U said she could not help me, which was an answer in itself. I declared that I dare not leave Alex.

There were already doctors thinking the effort had gone on too long. We were heading towards that decision and I felt the burden of the overwhelming challenge to me personally, but Dr U stated the decision about giving up would not be mine. I felt this moribund situation was emotionally between Alex and me and I changed to not wanting to share conversation about the son I had brought into the world with Alex's carers. I was unsure how I could talk to my family. Serena came towards the end of this chat from Dr U and I felt she needed not to be part of this.

I tried to explain to Dr S that we had fought so hard for Alex over the previous 5 years as I wanted them to understand Alex's state immediately prior to admission to ICU was not what I was saying Alex should live for. But it just seemed so hard for those seeing Alex now to understand what we could have kept working towards if we did not have this setback. Dr S looked doubtful about whether I should have introduced the topic at all. He said, "Let's just focus on what we have here and now". He was telling me, indirectly, that there was no hope in his view so I did not persist. They did not understand my fears that doctors might not regard Alex's life as worth living from the outset.

I had protected my family from the day by day anguish of Alex's admission and much of his previous day to day trials. I felt even more alone, as if my new state of mind could not be articulated and not understood by anyone. There was no escape, no luxury of withdrawing to an isolated spot to process the disaster. I just tried to hide the worst of the fears from anyone I had to talk to for a few days, including relatives in Melbourne. That night I rang Alex's father to tell him that things were grim, still minimising drama. I asked him if he would he be able to visit Alex knowing he had mobility problems and travel was difficult. He said he would try.

I removed permission for Alex's support coordinator and Serena to obtain information about Alex from the hospital. I told them of this change, trying to explain this was not personal.

Days 33 and 34 were spent with the gloom worsening. I tried explaining to Dr U the same things that I had tried with Dr S. Dr U listened more but I could see it was all too late. Dr U understood the issue of wanting not to lose Alex but not wanting him to suffer with a poor quality of life. I said he was already suffering. I had to dry tears so Alex would not see me knowing the worst. I expressed my despair that I was unskilled for what was now an excruciating role for me.

There was no way through the minefield. With NMS, Alex was very sick overall. Because of the intubation for his surgery followed by pneumonia combined with his distress on removal of sedation, independence from the breathing machine was delayed. With every delay the situation worsened. With a tracheostomy, things were a hundred-fold worse even if it was done originally with the intention of getting him to breathe on his own. With the removal of antipsychotics in order to attempt recovery from the NMS, the chances of recuperation, even if the slim chance recovery was achieved, were next to impossible. With his mental illness and other disabilities, he was not going to be able to live any kind of community life. In the worst-case scenario, if surviving, he would remain on a breathing machine with florid psychoses. I am not sure at what point in these weeks the aim of him breathing on his own was lost irretrievably.

The idea to use support workers 24/7 to help to keep Alex calm and diverted, when his sedation was eased, was slow to come to fruition because we needed a final OK from the hospital, and then Serena needed to allow time for responses from any previous workers available for shifts again. I do not think the hospital understood that workers were not just hanging about ready to come at short notice. A schedule of workers commenced but not until Day 37. The evening and night shifts were first to fill. The day shifts could not be filled so I took those, which at least meant I did not have to wait for normal visiting hours to be with Alex. Serena filled other gaps personally. The few workers able to come did a great job.

Day 35 Dr W was on duty for the weekend. His body language and tone were all pessimistic. He asked me about the photo on the poster of Alex being on his feet at the theatre. He wanted to know when was it and why he had needed a walker. He wrote 8 February next to the photo. Apparently, the physiotherapist had told everyone that Alex had been an invalid prior to his admission! This physiotherapist had met me in Alex's room and called me "Dear". On the second reference I said my name is not Dear, it is Helen. I do not think he understood my objection to his condescension. He also apparently did not listen properly to my story. When I told him Alex had only recently wanted the walker and it was not because of lack of strength in his legs, rather it was because of his fear of falling with the strange blank outs. Previously he had lots of energy and was a good walker, often charging ahead of others. How is this translated into him having invalid status? This was important because such ICU doctors give themselves the target of getting the patient back to pre-admission health and capabilities. Was this really further evidence for the argument that Alex's case was hopeless?

I spoke to my second son Ewen on Saturday Day 35. He wanted to fly from Hobart so I would not have to deal with this on my own. I told him to wait. Then, I was given better news about Alex's breathing and oxygen requirements in the next twenty-four hours. I relayed this better news to Ewen. It proved a very temporary hope.

Day 36 ICU again tried to move Alex to a chair but he found it very distressing. Day 37 Alex was upset a lot. We introduced his joke books which had needed to be found in the packed boxes of his belongings. He loved them and it was good to have them on hand. Staff had his Youtube connection permanently on tinkling calming music. Serena and I tried to include his favourites when we visited such as Michael Jackson and John Farnham. Serena also found the film Ghostbusters one night when she visited so they could share one of his favourite movies.

Alex's chest X-ray was bad on Day 38, worse than previously according to Dr U. He had another infection and a collapsed lung. This was a huge blow for Dr U as well as us because they knew this setback was going to make it impossible to keep arguing for the effort with Alex's machine. There were not going to be any further options.

Ewen flew from Hobart the next day and when he visited Alex looked worried. It was probably a shock to suddenly have a brother visit. We asked Alex if he wanted Ewen to stay. Squeeze my hand if yes. He squeezed my hand!

Ewen was in time for the dreaded meeting with Dr U. He held my hand while we were told the end would come this week. Dr U explained about timing within the uncertainties while in palliative care. They proposed waiting before removal of the tracheostomy so that family could say goodbye, and this was the plan we followed. Nonetheless I worried the whole time that we were keeping Alex suffering for this to occur, for others' benefit.

It was time to tell Serena, which Ewen and I did together by phone that evening. Shock and grief. Serena had given her heart and soul to having the best care possible for Alex in community and had learnt to love him in a short time.

Surrounded by family

Alex's father and other brothers came on Day 40. Alex took it all in with fears I could only guess at. He was awake enough to know and appreciate his visitors but could not communicate any dread he felt. He cried several times which was not his normal reaction to distress, even to pain. We cancelled the support workers. Ewen and Donald stayed with Alex all night. The joke books were a success. Alex gave belly laughs even though other communication was impossible. Alex's father had to be supported to walk in to the ward and get up from chairs. He could not stay long in Alex's room but at least he came.

I was not happy that Dr T was back on duty. I did not see Dr U again. I felt Dr T had discounted Alex already, even though he was still supported by the breathing machine and still very much in need of emotional support. Dr T would come to the door beckoning me for different matters, ignoring Alex and ignoring whatever interaction I might have been having with Alex at the time. I saw my main role was to be very present for Alex, not to satisfy Dr T's sense of immediacy to tell me something.

With Ewen, Donald and Clive doing a fantastic job supporting Alex and saintly nurses jollying him along, I felt better about going in and out to attend to the business side of the process. I was focussed, seeing time slow down to put my best foot forward, but I was becoming more and more tense. I was not detached. I kept postponing contact with undertakers despite a reminder from Nurse Experience.

There was some confusion over the palliative care arrangements. Alex would gradually die once the breathing machine was removed, with timing unknown. A couple of palliative care people came to meet with me in the small lounge. They clarified that Alex would not be moved to a separate palliative care ward, but ICU staff would be under their guidance from the time of removal of the breathing machine. Ewen and I had told ICU that scaring Alex with a move to the palliative care ward would be horrible in any case. I was assured Alex would be made comfortable. I asked about his potential for feeling distressed by the urge to breathe but not being able to get his lungs to work. I was told that there is "a drug" to be given to reduce or stop the breathing reflex.

Dr T arranged another meeting in the small lounge meeting room. Also in attendance was a nurse whom I had not met and a registrar with whom I had had intermittent contact over the weeks. He had been the one who asked me a couple of weeks earlier in front of Alex if Alex was a smoker. *Had they not worked that out yet?* I joked with him, "No, Alex would be the one telling him at length about the evils of smoking if he could talk". Alex smiled. This registrar had been present at the palliative care meeting also.

Dr T wanted to repeat what I had already heard from Dr U and from the palliative team. I attended on my own. I listened for any further details. He nodded at the nurse present. "She" will take out the tracheostomy in the morning. "She!?" I said, "Surely she has a name". I turned to the nurse to ask her name which she gave quietly, reserved in such a meeting. I did not want nurses to be treated as lesser workers nor did I want someone performing such an important role in Alex's life to be nameless. I was able to thank her directly at the end of her shift the next day.

I asked about the "drug" that would remove the desire to breathe. He said, "Well, that is the morphine, which we had already discussed would be used for pain and sedation". I looked across at the registrar wondering why he did not say this previously. I kept quiet, but it was another example of the importance of using drug names not just generic terms of drug or medicine or using the term bug for a bacterium in order to make sense of the conversations in hospital. They otherwise seemed to set aside quite a bit of time to make sure you knew what was happening.

When I was back with Alex, Dr T's finger beckoned me from Alex's door again. He brought me to the middle of the ICU area and with his registrar shadow told me there would be interest in organ donation from such a young man as Alex. The challenges kept coming. I was going to face whatever had to be faced. I said I had always agreed in principle with organ donation and would agree to an opportunity to help others. I decided to keep this latest challenge from the rest of the family as they had enough to deal with. A bit later Dr T said something about how Donate Australia might not use Alex considering the lack of oxygen but they would meet with me later. I was given a time of 5.30 to which I agreed.

I ruminated all afternoon on whether I was acting responsibly so when I had the opportunity to speak to Nurse Experience I reached out. I told her what Dr T had said and I had two questions. I wanted to know about the limitations on choosing Alex for organ donation and whether there would be any impulse to hasten his death for the organs. She doubly reassured me there were strict legal matters and protocols controlling organ donation. They would let him die of natural causes.

I met with Ewen in the waiting area shortly after 5pm for an update on everything. He said he wanted a family meeting shortly. I then admitted I had the meeting with Donate Australia. He was not upset and said he also agreed with the principle of offering help to others from organ donation. 5.30 pm came and went as did 6.30 pm. Nurse Experience passed, checked on us and went away to sort it out. It was after 7.00 pm before I had a meeting with Donate Australia, to which she also came to support me. The representative asked me what I knew and had been thinking. I noted my support for organ donation but said there were several things I could imagine preventing Alex from being a donor.

The representative told me Alex was not suitable. Not only was she able to reassure me that Alex would in no way be regarded as a suitable donor, but that there were processes that they normally follow before any such suggestion is made to relatives. They do research and assessments, with an informed decision to take to relatives. I said Dr T needed to be educated. I said he had not destabilised me but it was potentially very harmful. I held it together but it could have been so distressing that I would not have been a support to Alex or to anyone else in the family. Insensitive. I hoped he was not teaching bad habits to his registrar. They articulated that my comments would be taken "on board".

Ewen and Donald slept in fits and starts in Alex's room but tried to be awake whenever Alex was awake. They kept him amused with music and games on their devices. And by reading jokes of course.

We were all there by around 9 am on Day 41 and Serena came to say goodbye to Alex about 9.30 am. Ewen's wife flew in to be with us. Serena's tears flowed freely and Alex concentrated on her face. He valued her being there but I grew anxious because none of us was indicating there was no hope. Alex let Serena go without too much distress thankfully. I had been telling him he had been very sick but he had good doctors and nurses and we were trying to get him better. Was this a loving and moral thing to keep up in his final hours? The boys and I had agreed that we would all take this approach. I will not know whether it would have been better for me, like Serena, to have given recognition to the fear of death that Alex must have held at that moment, and cried with him.

I had to give the signal we were ready for the tracheostomy to be removed. Extra sedation. Specialists abounding. The nurse doing the removal entered. Very carefully they began. Alex found it distressing. I got close to him and looked him in the eye. "It is alright Alex", I said using reassuring tones and caresses. The real story is you are about to die my precious son. I felt like a traitor or at least a con-artist but thought it was my role for his needs nonetheless. I had so often told him I would never lie to him. I wanted the inevitable to be as comfortable for him as possible of course but was I discounting his wishes?

With the tube in his throat removed, but with oxygen tubing to his nose, he was surviving using his own breathing, even if laboured. The day was spent attending to the wound from the hole in his throat, keeping him comfortable attending to for example the mucous build ups, still with monitoring of his vital signs. Alex was being given more and more morphine.

Was Alex going to surprise them all and really breathe on his own? Of course I was deluded to entertain such thoughts. *Were they going to sedate him so much it would be impossible to achieve that?* I was trusting them with Alex's last hours in their hands to get the right balance to let him go with minimal suffering. It had been six weeks of a fine balancing act.

During the afternoon, Nurse Experience took me for a constitutional around the hospital grounds. "Just to get you out of this environment for a bit", she said. It was nice to spend a half hour chatting as two humans rather than as a nurse and family of a patient. I told her I did not necessarily trust the hospital to call us in time if we abandoned our watch on Alex. I told her of my experience when my mother died. We left her very ill at the hospital and when they did ring, she had already died.

Following the all-night vigil, Ewen needed a rest in the afternoon but Donald soldiered on. By Friday evening it was clear that we were not going to go the distance for Alex without taking rest breaks. I did not want my other sons getting sick. If I had said I would stay, the others would not want me to be on my own so would not rest. Once Alex seemed settled and asleep by about 8.30 pm, we all left. Perhaps he was unconscious and never going to wake. We sought assurances from staff that we would be contacted should Alex wake.

I was suddenly woken by a call on my phone at about 3 am on Day 42. I recognised Dr S's voice. "I am sorry to call in the middle of the night but Alex's death is imminent." "We are about ten minutes away and we will be there", I said carefully. I rushed to wake the others. Alex's father felt he could not attend with us and he had seen Alex the previous day to say goodbye.

The road was closed for night roadworks! We had to spend an extra fifteen minutes seeking out an alternative route in an unfamiliar area. We could only do what we could do. There was a further delay at the hospital entrance with uncertainty about whether we should be using the Emergency Department entrance which is a hike round the corner. After a phone call, an ICU nurse came down to open the front door.

On entering ICU Dr S stopped me to prepare me for Alex's current state. Yes, he was awake as far as his current sedation would allow, as much as you could call it awake. He warned me that Alex was already suffering from insufficient oxygen and was going blue. His brain would have been damaged such that he would not be able to respond to me.

We spent the next two hours with Alex who was gasping. Each breathe was noisy and agonising. His eyes were open but he was not seeing. His mouth was in an "O". We held his hands. Nurse Experience told us to keep talking to Alex. I cradled his head in my arms as far as I could reach. Towards the end a nurse asked me if I wanted the bed down. I shook my head more from not wanting anything to interrupt my attention on

Alex than from not wanting to get closer. I was frozen in watching and waiting.

Sedation was changed several times in dosing and administration. Subcutaneous rather than in line was going to get faster action. Every now and then a nurse poked her head in.

I could feel him getting colder. After all those weeks of having a raised temperature!

"I am your mum and you are my son. I am always your mum. I am always with you."

I had my cheek on his forehead. The rhythm of his breathing changed. There was a pause so I moved to see his face. He gasped again so I held him against me again. Another pause and I knew there were no more breaths. I cried out, not needing to be calm anymore.

I wailed from a hilltop to all. "No More! They cannot hurt you anymore!"

I think I was half sobbing and half gasping. Nurse Experience came to tell me to take deep breaths. I acceded and steadied myself and went round the family checking they were OK. This was beyond their experiences. I took a last look into Alex's face and resisted the temptation to close his eyes.

Alex was too big to be taken to the morgue so he had to be taken directly by an undertaker. Now I needed to select someone quickly. My sons searched and we made the call. I was given a last goodbye to Alex.

I went to the opposite side from where I had cradled him. I touched his arm and promised we would keep looking after him. We would do our very best.

Part 2 The issues needing attention

What is to be done?

Change is required for those with the dual disabilities. While the Royal Commission into Violence, Abuse, Neglect and Exploitation of People with a Disability[12] made valuable recommendations, Alex's story points to additional recommendations. The recommendations I have drafted in this part have not been refined yet with other stakeholders and interested parties, and should be seen as starting points.

Improvement targets are divided into three categories:

1. The foremost issues dealing with human rights and discrimination in diagnosis and treatment. If the doctors that everyone look up to and rely on cannot get it right, there is no hope for anything else in the system to work
2. The auxiliary issues attached to the mental health system where additional mistakes, such as failure to use others who know the patient, exacerbate the worsening state or lack of recovery, and
3. The issues associated with the need for health to work with the community – the interface with disability services and housing for example.

---

[12] The pertinent recommendations from the Royal Commission into Violence, Abuse, Neglect and Exploitation of People with a Disability are from Volume 6 (Enabling autonomy and access) of the Final Report (September 2023). Section 4.3 *Health System* gives a description of the actions being taken to improve health services for those with cognitive disabilities, including through the National Roadmap. The Royal Commission's many recommendations are in the right direction but need to be implemented.

355

1. The foremost issues

Denial of Human Rights

People with a disability should receive nothing less than the standard of treatment and services received by those without a disability.

Alex's human rights were denied in several different circumstances. This was influenced by the fear of his behaviour and presumption of criminality, irrational denial of need for health care, shifting of responsibility or willingness to justify the lack of use of limited resources in his complex case.

His human rights were denied when held legally in involuntary admission to a health facility, if it were not in the least restrictive manner possible.

Alex's rights to mental health services were denied by those who could not look past his cognitive disabilities to contemplate his mental illness. His human right to mental health services were also denied when clinicians treated him without taking cognitive disability into account in their manner of assessment. This was a path to inadequate care through not adjusting communication and interpretations. If your mindset is based on negative discrimination, then human rights are forgotten.

The relevant specific incidents are listed in the following table.

Experience	Specific incidents	Text
Hospitals/GP in rejecting Alex's access to care	Canberra Hospital admitted Alex for only two weeks in 2017 and discharged him without proper assessment, without a discharge plan and after removal of one of his critical medicines.	Ch 4
	Victorian Large Regional Hospital was determined that Alex never be admitted there regardless of presentation.	Ch 11
	After initially accepting him as a patient Victorian local GP banned Alex with disregard for the acute help he needed.	Ch 12
Housing ACT rejecting rights to accommodation even when supported by others	After stating in writing that Alex was eligible for housing in 2018, by 2021 we were told Alex could not be given public housing. Housing's rationale for turning their earlier decision around was never entirely clear. Its defence was loosely based on his lack of independence, but this would bar every person who needed family or disability worker	Ch 10

	supports. Housing belatedly admitted they were scared off by the behaviour specialist's report painting Alex at his worst while inadequately medicated. There seemed to be a justification for loss of rights once it was assumed Alex was at his baseline state for that assessment.	
Nurse lack of professionalism: laughing at distress, use of physical force, remaining aloof	Alex's rights were compromised by being in an inappropriate institution with staff not trained to cope. Staff lost respect as a first professional principle. Some of the nurses at Dhulwa developed a manipulative routine of taunting Alex and then laughing at him when he reacted. With his preoccupation about his things not to be interfered with, they would threaten to go to his room as a controlling tool.	Ch 9
	I personally observed a nurse physically hold Alex down on a visit to Dhulwa when he had not done anything physically	Ch 7

	threatening. Calling security guards to menace Alex, if not restrain him, was commonplace.	
	Another tool from nurses which denied human rights was refusal to engage, remaining aloof when he might have wanted friendly conversation. Many nurses could not see the benefit of developing a human relationship. It seemed to be patient blaming.	Ch 11
	Alex's lack of access to normal personal care such as getting a haircut also meant he could not retain dignity. Doctors recorded his appearance as unkempt as if it was part of his normal clinical features.	Ch 10
Nurse breaches of confidentiality: giving patient information to external parties	Nurses forgot their patients' rights in their bid to meet a desperate agenda about fear of assault from several patients. Alex was included in the release of confidential information to unauthorised parties and to insecure systems such as their home emails. This occurred at the time of Alex's rebound	Epilogue Ch10

	mental illness after his first episode of neuroleptic malignant syndrome when he could have been extremely frightening to unprepared nurses.	
Hospital breach of confidentiality with community, including police	In 2022, the large Regional Hospital in Victoria revealed information about Alex to a non-family member (my landlord), prospective community organisations and Small Town police. My permission was not sought. The landlord and the police had their own interests at heart, not Alex's.	Ch 12
Fallback to indefinite detention or delay	Dhulwa's fallback position on managing Alex in the face of opposition from the ACT police to allow him in the community was to have no plan forward. Dhulwa preferred to lock him up indefinitely with no new treatments or programs.	Ch 8
Pushing discharge when failure would be assured from untreated mental illness: reputational	Rights to health care were repeatedly absent. At the beginning of his last five years Alex was pushed out of Canberra Hospital with not just lack of assessment but with harm done through	Chs 4-12

damage and opportunities lost	clinical sloppiness. During his ensuing tortured years, discussions about his future were hampered or went in circles while hospitals pushed for discharge against a community not able to support him. The Regional Hospital in Victoria went further, in trying to push him into their own community arrangements without representative consent or even acknowledging me and with rude claims of his carers dumping Alex for no clinical reason at the hospital.	
Community infringement of rights to privacy and fair process in pursuit of rage against disability residency in community	Small Town's perceptions about their own rights blinded residents to Alex's rights. They aired antagonism about having an SDA built in the middle of Small Town and having Alex reside there. It was very suspicious that residents thought they knew Alex's medical information and NDIS funding. They had no legal right to prevent Alex from living there.	Ch 13

Discrimination against those with cognitive problems within mental health services.

An aversion to seeing the medical needs of someone with cognitive disability is compounded when the problem is mental illness, when the symptoms can be brushed away as due to disability and not due to treatable conditions. The Australian Government Department of Health Capability Framework[13] calls for professionals to employ appropriate assessment procedures and tools to inform diagnosis of health conditions, with an awareness that modified diagnostic criteria and reasonable adjustments may be required for assessment of people with intellectual disability. Equity in outcomes is not achieved through treating everyone the same.[14]

Discrimination also occurs when a psychiatrist cannot see beyond cognitive disability. There seem to be too many psychiatrists who approach their work with a blindness to mental illness once they perceive cognitive disability. There are none so blind as those who will not see. This blindness is described as systemic and wilful ignorance in a submission to

---

[13] https://www.health.gov.au/resources/publications/intellectual-disability-health-capability-framework?language=en

[14] A case report about someone with cerebral palsy seeking health care supplied to the Royal Commission (Volume 6, page 349) succinctly made the same point, "not treating him differently meant not treating him appropriately". *Royal Commission into Violence, Abuse, Neglect and Exploitation of People with Disability (September, 2023). This material is referenced under a Creative Commons Attribution 4.0 International licence (www.creativecommons.org/licenses).*

the Royal Commission into Violence, Abuse, Neglect and Exploitation of People with a Disability[15]

I was suspicious that Alex's experiences of discrimination were an effort to cost-shift to the disability sector. It was difficult to find any dissenting doctors not affected by group-think on the issue. The rejection of Alex as a patient by the Regional Hospital could have been affected by, not only their lack of expertise in handling the psychiatric needs of a person with cognitive disability, but also by a general desire to push those with a cognitive disability into the disability care sector away from their own responsibilities.

Time and again in Alex's last five years he experienced diagnostic overshadowing. Why are psychiatrists stuck in this paradigm? Better diagnostic methods is not new thinking and can be traced to work earlier than that of the Royal Commission. [16]

Towards the end of his life, Alex was not in the best circumstances for care of his physical needs either.

---

[15] Submission to the Royal Commission into Violence, Abuse, Neglect and Exploitation of People with a Disability by Dr Jennifer Torr, Consultant Psychiatrist specialising in the psychiatry of old age and the psychiatry of intellectual disability.

[16] For example, the research on this topic to 2014 was summarised for the lay person in a short article in The Conversation[16] by a collaboration from Warwick UK and Monash Australia universities, 12 November 2014. The Authors, R Hastings, B Tonge, G Melvin, K Gray and V Totsika noted that better methods were required for diagnosis of mental illness in those with intellectual disabilities, recognising early intervention as all important.

Incidents of discrimination in mental health systems because of Alex's cognitive problems are:

Experience	Specific incidents	Text
Diagnostic overshadowing: lack of interest in mental illness once patient seen to have intellectual disabilities	Dr B was emphatic that Alex had intellectual disability and therefore was not to be admitted to a mental health unit. Becoming aware that this was a mistake and recommencing antipsychotics did not mean all would be well. Multiple doctors thereafter were insistent, once they could see antipsychotics addressing some of Alex's problems, that the remainder were due to Intellectual disability and were therefore not their responsibility. The Victorian Regional Hospital as reported above had a fixation that Alex did not have mental illness. It looked very much as if this bias was amplified as Alex progressed from one	Ch 4 Ch 12 Ch13

	health service to another through Alex's transfer notes. It was possible that Dhulwa was instrumental in ensuring everybody assumed that Alex behaviours were not due to mental illness as he was being given an antipsychotic.	
Failure to adapt psychiatric reviews given intellectual disabilities	Alex's representative should have been included as was sometimes happening at the Adult Mental Health Unit, but not at Dhulwa, possibly because it was a locked facility, and only with difficulty in Victoria. I can only guess at what methods were used; what adaptation of questioning was employed. I have the evidence of failure to see manic symptoms as evidence of poor adaptability of methods.	Chs 8-9
Failure to consider different presentation possibilities when dual diagnosis present	Nurses persistently believed that manic symptoms were displays of Alex's childlike play-acting arising from his cognitive problems	Ch 4

Application of discipline designed for normal intellect such as denial of activities otherwise appropriate to be considered for preventing aggression	Dhulwa applied its disciplinary approach inflexibly, with DASA scores for example, consistent with its approach to other patients. It discriminated against Alex because he was least able to exhibit the control required given his lack of appropriate medication and his need for rituals. It denied him therapeutic activities on a spurious model.	Ch 7

Clinical mismanagement

There were so many health professional mistakes or examples of poor practice in Alex's last five years. Of most significance is the way he was treated in the Adult Mental Health Unit Canberra Hospital with Dr B a particular offender. This is significant because it launched his five-year horror story and progression to early death. Once his mental health was so compromised by failures to properly medicate him, his "norm" was documented to include certain alarming behaviours with no understanding of a better Alex, and each subsequent phase was downhill. His worsening mental health reduced anyone's ability to care for his physical health.

How could the psychiatrists of Canberra's Acute Mental Health Unit be so adamant that Alex did not suffer from mental illness? Did they believe that intellectual disability precluded mental illness or perhaps that the two could not occur together? Were they so anxious to limit use of their resources that they latched onto Alex's cognitive problems to find an excuse not to treat him? How did they not take account of all that he had been through in diagnoses and treatments up to that point of his life at 35 years?

You would have thought that professionals would be aware that mental illness is frequently found concurrently with cognitive disabilities, so it should not have been a strange concept. There was evidence presented to the Royal Commission into Violence, Abuse, Neglect and Exploitation of People with a Disability about high rates of mental health conditions among people with cognitive disability[17].

There was a study using Western Australian data from registers for each of intellectual disability and psychiatric

---

[17] Professor Julian Trollor reported to the Royal Commission: "Best estimates suggest that for common disorders such as schizophrenia, affective and anxiety disorders and dementias, prevalence in people with intellectual disability is 2 to 3 times that of the general population ...".
During Public hearings 4 and 6 of the Royal Commission into Violence, Abuse, Neglect and Exploitation of People with a Disability it heard from several witnesses about barriers to quality mental health care and treatment faced by people with cognitive disability.
Royal Commission into Violence, Abuse, Neglect and Exploitation of People with Disability (September 2023). This material is referenced under a Creative Commons Attribution 4.0 International licence (www.creativecommons.org/licenses).

disorders by Morgan et al (2008)[18]. They found that almost a third of individuals with intellectual disability had concurrent psychiatric morbidity. They also acknowledged that this is probably an underestimate because of poor diagnostic capabilities. How many of those with dual disability are poorly diagnosed and struggle for access to mental health care like Alex did, despite this relatively high likelihood based on prevalence? How widespread is the culture of assigning undesirable behaviours to non-mental illness conditions called 'behaviours'?

Aggression can form part of a mental illness. There has been some research into violent or aggressive behaviours linked to bipolar disorder or mania. For example, Gonzalez-Ortega et al. (2010)[19] revealed a relationship between lack of insight by the patient to their mental illness and aggressive behaviour during acute mania occasioning involuntary admission to hospital. Ballester et al. (2012)[20] compared those with any history of bipolar disorder, non-bipolar psychopathology and healthy controls. They concluded that those with bipolar disorder experience greater rates of aggression, especially during acute and psychotic episodes. Care in the refined diagnosis and thus

---

[18] Morgan V A, Leonard H, Bourke J and Jablensky A (2008) Intellectual disability co-occurring with schizophrenia and other psychiatric illness: population-based study The British Journal of Psychiatry 193, 364-372. doi:10.1192/bjp.107.044461.

[19] Gonzalez-Ortega I, Mosquera F, Echeburua E and Gonzalez-Pinto A (2010) Insight, psychosis and aggressive behaviour in mania Eur. J. Psychiat. 24(2):70-77.

[20] Ballester J, Goldstein T, Goldstein B, Obreja M, Axelson D, et al. (2012) Is bipolar disorder specifically associated with aggression? Bipolar Disord.:14(3):283-290. (NIH Public Access)

the appropriate treatment of Alex's range of symptoms was important.

Some specific examples of poor practice in the mental health facilities responsible for Alex.

Experience	Specific incidents	Text
Failure to make provisions for day-to-day hygiene and physical care where patient unable to provide for himself	Alex contracted cellulitis in August 2018, possibly because of bacterial entry with feet fungal infections. His sheets and towels were never washed. He possibly commenced his lack of personal washing at this stage. There was no assistance for Alex, assuming he could look after himself.	Ch 5
Failure to read manic symptoms – a repeated theme	In 2017, the poor judgement in removing clozapine was compounded by neither nurses nor psychiatrists detecting Alex's subsequent emergent manic symptoms and delusions, which if seen at all, were accepted as play from someone with an intellectual disability.	Ch 4

	Residual manic symptom observations repeatedly reported by me were ignored during 2018. No one was accepting that Alex was not adequately treated by the olanzapine, risperidone etc. tried during 2018.	Ch 5
	In 2022, the responsible Victorian community mental health service would not recognise manic symptoms saying Alex was autistic and needed time to settle.	Ch 11
Persistence with treatment regardless of evidence	The Adult Mental Health Unit Canberra Hospital refused for months to acknowledge that the antipsychotics tried after removing clozapine were inadequate for Alex.	Chs 4-5
	Dhulwa persisted with using clozapine only in 2022 on the argument that it was the "main one" and he did not have manic symptoms - all else was due to intellectual disability?	Ch 10
Group think from one service to	While we kept thinking that we had at last	Ch 14

another either from poor communications or single source credo	overcome the bias against Alex regarding his manic symptoms and need for additional psychiatric care, the persistence that it was just ID or autism emerged at the two last health services caring for him: Western Mental Health Services and ICU at Western Melbourne Hospital came up with this nonsense as if they had selectively read notes or had been verbally told to ignore Alex's mother.	
Lack of care on potential over-medication	Dhulwa discharged Alex on a very high dose of clozapine in 2022 with no explanation, and contrary to documented plans. No care seems to have been taken by any of the subsequent services to monitor the situation given Alex's first bout of NMS in January 2022. It was not until January 2023 that his clozapine blood levels were measured and found to be above therapeutic level. Higher	Ch 14

	doses can be a risk factor for NMS.	
Failure of follow up between facilities regarding dosing and monitoring of side effects	The prescribing of cariprazine by Dr O just as Alex was being discharged from the Regional Hospital was welcomed but ran foul with the lack of communications between services on a matter that should have been a high priority given the risks. An additional antipsychotic was being prescribed for someone who had contracted NMS the previous year. There was good reason to try cariprazine for the mania, but not without warning those subsequently caring for Alex. No effort was made to describe in handovers what the prescriber intended for ongoing adjustments of dose and what should be considered about the high dose of clozapine.	Chs 14-15
Failure to check patient's history regarding prescription of	Multiple doctors looked at Alex's OCD-like symptoms and said why don't we try sertraline, without ever	Chs 3, 4 and 15

drugs found useless or harmful previously e.g. to consider manic side effects of sertraline	tracing what happened when Alex was given that previously. Dhulwa prescribed sertraline without a concern for mania which they could/would not see. Even the psychiatrist at Western Melbourne Hospital in Alex's last days wanted to give Alex sertraline as supposedly some sort of control, should he have his sedatives removed while he also was not being treated with antipsychotics.	
Psychiatrist seen as infallible: despite responsibility to acquire advice when treating those with intellectual disability	There was a lack of leadership in securing relevant dual disability expertise for Dhulwa which had a culture of believing its skills were sufficient.	Ch 10
	Victorian Mental Health Service nearest to Small Town had to be nagged into seeking advice from the Victorian Dual Disability Service and then only used it superficially	Ch 11

	without giving it all the facts. Large Regional Hospital gave heavy reliance on a psychiatric assessment within the facility when that psychiatrist failed to involve the representative and appears to have only spoken with Alex while he was sedated. What information was he using?	Ch 12
Health administrators looking to other factors before clinical assessment and treatment risks	For example, Dhulwa's review excluded what was happening with their psychiatrists and omitted questioning how appropriately skilled they were for those such as Alex. Throughout most of the horror story, the clinical contributions were not questioned by anyone in the team inside or outside the service, until the Behaviour Specialist (Victoria) could see what was happening in Small Town with Alex and what the mental health service was not doing - a stark	Preface

	situation that medical people could not see.	

Recommendations

1. Raise awareness within health facilities that disabilities should not compromise human rights afforded those without disabilities. Enforce administrative codes of practice in effecting human rights principles. All mental health professionals have a responsibility to provide quality mental health care to their clients, including those with an intellectual disability (Article 25 of the United National Convention on the Rights of Persons with Disabilities). There seems to be a need to augment professional training on the rights of those with disabilities. Wide use of the Capability Framework is to be supported.

2. Increase resources to mental health care so that any pressure to override human rights is removed. Resources should be sufficient for allocation of extra specialist time or a specialist team to consider complex cases.

3. Improve Psychiatric training. Emphasise the increased likelihood that people with an intellectual disability also have a mental illness. Increase understanding about the presentations resulting from this dual disability. Training should involve an understanding of how the two disabilities work together and not as necessarily separate conditions to be divided for administrative reasons. Training should include preparation for handling reviews and assessment of mentally

ill patients with cognitive issues, involving the approach, questions asked and analysis of responses. Anti-bias training is also required. Resources such as the Intellectual Disability Mental Health Core Competency Framework Manual[21] and associated toolkit which has been available since 2016 should be used by those working in mental health with those with intellectual disabilities.

Attention to the training of psychiatrists, neurologists and paediatricians on cross-disease aetiologies is required. Greater understanding of the similar pathophysiological pathways behind intellectual disability, developmental delay, autism, epilepsy, schizophrenia and Tourette's syndrome is emerging[22].

4. Explore the required Specialist mental health facilities, either as a stand-alone specialist unit, or as part of a larger general facility which includes staff with training in the notion of discipline of those with cognitive impairment and in behaviour support. There is some evidence for better

---

21

https://www.3dn.unsw.edu.au/sites/default/files/IDMH_Core_Co mpetency_Framework.pdf.
https://www.3dn.unsw.edu.au/sites/default/files/IDMH_Core_Co mpetency_Framework_Toolkit.pdf.

[22] Given the considerable evidence, we propose a reasonable hypothesis that these (neurodevelopmental) diseases may have a common network of pathogenesis, and Ash1l may be located at the epicentre hub of neural co-networks that are the centre of pathological damage. Found in DOI: 10.1002/dneu.22795 REVIEW ARTICLE Role of Ash1l in Tourette syndrome and other neurodevelopmental disorders Cheng Zhan, Lulu Xu, Xueping Zheng, Shiguo Liu and Fengyuan Che *Developmental Neurobiology.* 2021;81:79–91.

outcomes in intellectual disability specialist mental health services (Melvin et al., 2022)[23]. These facilities should also recognise the additional personal care that might be required for hygiene and preventive health care. They should have processes for cross-checking diagnoses with independent experts of mental illness patients with cognitive impairment.

5. Determine reasons for mindsets and group think so they can rectify any systemic or professional contributors to failures to consider more than what appeared in a previous report as part of system administration.

6. Allow time for medical personnel to reflect on how much they rely on an existing report or referral even when the medical area is contentious, the patient may exhibit idiosyncratic symptoms and so much is still being learnt on the subject.

7. Investigate failures of a service or facility to adequately and in a timely way pick up the care of transferred mental health patients. Each new mental health care provider should first be aware of the urgencies associated with the new patient care. Victoria showed that this is carelessly done, whether from hospital to community mental health care or from one regional mental care unit to another.

8. Require consultant psychiatrists to keep up to date on the research about diseases such as schizophrenia which is still not

---

[23] Melvin C, Barnoux M, Alexander R, Roy A, Devrapriam J, Blair R, Tromans S, Shepstone L and Langdon P E (2022) A systematic review of in-patient psychiatric care for people with intellectual disabilities and/or autism: effectiveness, patient safety and experience. British Journal of Psychiatry Open 8, e187, 1-18. doi: 10.1192/bjo.2022.571.

fully understood and whose presentation can vary from person to person. Pharmacological treatments need to be better understood in relation to variances in symptoms and presentations.

9. Include the potential for diagnostic overshadowing and prevalence of relevant qualifications to be able to discriminate diagnostic possibilities when determining the scope of reviews of systems and facilities.

10. Require the Chief Psychiatrist and Directors of Psychiatry to take the lead in an open evaluation of whether the clinical staff at a facility meet the purpose of the facility, especially to first do no harm.

2. Auxiliary issues

Failure to use guardian/representative

Information transfer from me and to me should have been happening but was neglected or deliberately curtailed. Information sharing with discussions was almost impossible.

Conducting reviews and interviews without the patient's representative being present compromised care and ignored the patient's rights to participate even if through a representative. Assessments were at risk of being based on misinterpretations and incomplete information. Staff were effectively keeping Alex in ignorance if not relaying information to the representative on what tests are being conducted, what results are being obtained, and what rationales are for the treatment regime.

Victoria was bad overall in using me as a spokesperson and interpreter for Alex. There seemed to be a culture of ignoring representatives as if involving them was only a dispensable option. What contact I had with the Mental Health Service for Small Town was hampered by the ear plugs all staff seemed to put in place when I spoke, or the blindfold to my emails. The Regional Hospital wanted to pretend I did not exist for Alex's arrangements and care which it wanted to control and dictate.

Dhulwa in the ACT did not involve me in any of the doctor's sessions with Alex, whereas the Adult Mental Health Unit did. I interpreted this as meaning Dhulwa rejected my involvement because of their rules about not taking outsiders near patients unless they had training for safety. No attempt was made to find a room away from other patients but to which Alex and I could be present together. Dhulwa nominally used me by inviting me to Alex's Individual Care Plan meetings which were exercises in creating documents, not in guiding action.

After five years, when I begged to be listened to, with a figurative megaphone, and backing my arguments with more explicit descriptions of Alex's dire state, I was still ignored. When my daughter-in-law co-wrote with me seeking help, we were ignored. Family information was apparently a waste of their time.

All my submissions in making complaints in the ACT and Victoria and to government representatives came to nothing.

Experience	Specific incidents	Text
Failures to get history from representative and discounting representative credibility	When Alex was first admitted to Canberra Hospital in November 2017, I was invited to talk with the assessing psychiatrist. This should have been good, but he chose to ignore the all-important information about aripiprazole, leading to disaster.	Ch 4
	The worst example was at Victorian Large Regional Hospital which said, using its psychiatrist's assessment, that Alex did not have	Ch 12

	mental illness (despite the manic symptoms etc). That psychiatrist made no attempt to contact me for context. Once that assessment had been made, a defensive social worker said the psychiatrist could only go on the information he had. So whose fault was it that he had limited information?	
Failure to check documents written about Alex with representative at times when there was potential to misconstrue and be inaccurate	A Dhulwa staff member wrote up for file something that was supposed to be their background to his life. When I gave feedback that it had the wrong number of brothers for Alex and had things in his history skewed, I was ignored and again treated as if I should not help make sure their files were accurate. When I reported an Occupational Therapist report had errors, I was ignored and then told it could not be rectified because that staff member had left.	Ch 9
Hospital ignoring representative in	The Regional Hospital only contacted me when they	Ch 12

effort to seek accommodation while trying to get rid of patient after refusing care and removing representative from email trail (Large Regional Hospital)	wanted to manipulate a situation: 1. To set up blame for the support organisation 2. To pressure me into accepting that Alex could not be cared for by the Regional Health system. It excluded me from emails about arrangements and tried to override my authority to approve or not the proposals.	
Interpreting representative as cause of behaviour problems in patient	The Adult Mental Health Unit often wrote up their notes with me as the trigger for Alex's aggression. Some staff could not see that mothers can allow restraint collapse by their role as carer and comforter.	Ch 6

Patient blaming

The Capability Framework asks for professionals to treat all people with intellectual disability with dignity and respect, seeing them as a person first.

At first Dhulwa was resistant to the need for making changes to better care for Alex. I tried to promote behaviour support rather than behaviour management and to ask them to think

384

about what environmental changes might obviate some of his triggers. Of course, this was all working around the edges when he was inadequately diagnosed and poorly medicated.

Allied Health staff easily picked up on the view that Alex was a problem patient because of his intellectual disability. They reacted with the strategy that with discipline he could still be taught better behaviour. He was being naughty like a child, right? Alex was hard to manage and resentment built.

In addition, I seem to have been regarded as a problem mother/representative because I had not disciplined Alex. I had the temerity to resist the theory that they need not attend to his mental illness and kept trying to explain what Alex was like when optimally medicated. The allied health manager at the Canberra Hospital took on the role of managing me with a heavy-handed approach to try to get me to see their skewed views. The allied health manager at Dhulwa appointed as my liaison point, so that I would not annoy the doctors, was fixated on Alex having autism, which was a diagnosis that should have been qualified as not typical. She could not understand why I said Alex did not need pictures in their communications because he could read very well, and why I wanted justification for their training scheme for his autistic rituals.

Experience	Specific incidents	Text
Barriers to care from nurses and allied health.	I was not present for a lot of the interactions inside the facilities, but I surmised: Antagonism towards Alex	Chs 7-8

	because of aggression and violence. Stigma from his having 'behaviours' believing he was undisciplined, had bad parenting, and/or could be trained out of the behaviours such as with their meal discipline at Dhulwa. Ignorance of need to establish a relationship with Alex	
Admission to facility as deserved custodial sentence instead of therapeutic treatment	An acting senior staff member at Dhulwa asked me had I not been assaulted by Alex? She was implying that I should just accept his incarceration when, in contrast, I was looking for a new approach to Alex's mental health treatment.	Ch 7
Setting of impossible contracts to improve behaviour	Dhulwa put great emphasis on their discipline using DASA scores, taking ages to realise it was inappropriate for Alex. It never acknowledged it was counterproductive.	Ch 7
Emphasis on reactive measures (risk management rather than risk reduction or behaviour	It emerged in the series of Individual Care Plan meetings that the behaviour management to which Dhulwa was referring was about staff safety without	Ch 8

management instead of behaviour support)	components which would be therapeutic for Alex.

Failures of communication within the same health system

The ACT patient record system was fragmented in Alex's experience with lack of communication between the mental health databases and medical databases. Once a patient was moved into a medical area, as happened several times for Alex because of infections, doctors had to manually see his mental health notes and medication list. Maybe it has improved since Alex's time.

I describe in Chapter 3 how Alex's records could not be used to obtain a reliable history including medication types and dosages. There did not appear to be any checks on the accuracy and completeness of information inserted by the community mental health units.

The hospital assessing psychiatrist in November 2017 made a disastrous error in omitting aripiprazole saying it was not on his list as described. Where did he get that list? I know the same hospital could include aripiprazole on his medication list when he was admitted for cellulitis in 2014. Was it using a different database? What hospital records were they using in 2017? Was this psychiatrist using an old section of a mental health database? Why did he totally ignore me?

I needed to keep asking questions about what was happening with Alex. Apart from the diagnostic overshadowing, and the subsequent worsening of Alex's mental health, nurses could not be relied upon to make accurate and appropriate records for the doctors to read to make their decisions. Records were written up without understanding the symptoms being displayed (petit mal, mania and delusions) and with a view to downplay or upgrade Alex's aggression and outbursts as they saw fit.

I knew that communications within Dhulwa were poor when at Dhulwa meetings staff would give a supposed update on Alex which I knew was out of date because I would have spoken with Alex that morning, getting a different view.

I was not always told when Alex had shown bad behaviour, let alone why. I was not told the basis for decisions about leave, which might have been for reasons outside his behaviour but based on lack of staff, for example.

In Chapter 3, and other places, I noted that doctors could be loose in their language in making records. For example, many seem to like "historically violent" which, as I have discussed, is ambiguous. The result was that Alex's periods of lack of violence were never considered. No effort was made to link changes in Alex regarding aggression and violence with medication.

I wondered many times how anybody could get an accurate picture of a patient with the level of carelessness I saw in documentation.

Experience	Specific incidents	Text
Tightly held patient records by private practitioners	Records of medication tried could not be obtained from Alex's private psychiatrist, even when it was important for subsequent best clinical decisions.	Ch 2
Different record systems from one area of a hospital or health system to another.	The Emergency Department or medical wards could not open the mental health database and vice versa. Staff developed a work-around but the inefficiency and potential for error was obvious. There was another level of disconnection between mental health and medical wards when the nurses in the ward where Alex was taken on recovery form his first bout of NMS insisted on offering Alex Coloxyl (for constipation) when for the previous few days Alex had suffered from frequent faecal incontinence episodes once off clozapine. I know because I cleaned up most of them. "Dhulwa had charted the Coloxyl" was the excuse - while Alex was **on** clozapine.	Ch 6 and others

Incomplete medication histories and differences between sets of records	Hospital Progress Notes, crisis team reports and Clozapine Clinic notes for Alex differed in style and detail, gave no confidence that a complete history could be obtained. GP notes and private psychiatry would have to be added too. This would have been important for tracing what happened whenever Alex was given sertraline and answering questions about the value of valproate. Regardless, there was clearly a hospital record in the system that aripiprazole was included in Alex's regime in 2014, although denied by the hospital in 2017.	Ch 3
Setting up leave for essential external dentist with wording interpreted by others in manner at odds with intention	The Dhulwa Leave Committee set up a condition, which if not met, meant Alex could not attend a dental appointment. In the event he had not met the condition, but not for reasons predicting bad behaviour for an appointment. The important dental care was refused. No	Ch 9

	one was communicating rationally.	
Failure to undertake transfers with full communications from one health unit to another	Alex's transfer to Victoria, his transfer from Small Town to the Regional Hospital, the transfers back to community to two different mental health units in sequence were each handled badly with shocking lack or delay of proper care resulting. It might be simplistic to blame only a lack of good communication.	Ch 13

Recommendations

11. Fulsomely maintain patient records which should read in their entirety, not just scanned to see what matches biases and prejudiced conclusions. Staff should not make records for purposes other than to reflect what was observed.

12. Train all staff at a mental health facility and give refresher courses to increase understanding of mental illness, treated and untreated and ensure they are culturally attuned to seeing that patients are not to blame.

13. Educate staff caring for patients with coexistent cognitive problems, on the range and basic elements of the disabilities presented.

14. Remove the prevailing gospel that 'behaviours' not mental illness is appropriate just because the patient is complex with

cognitive problems. A culture change is required based on better understanding.

15. Train all staff in therapeutic approaches and strategies (such as behaviour support) as well as safety procedures and harm prevention.

16. Establish that a legal guardian/representative acts for the patient unable to take in all information and process it themselves so that they are included in doctor conversations with patients, and where that is impractical such as in a closed facility, a full report should be given to the representative who should then have an opportunity to respond and ask questions.

17. Use a guardian/representative and/or family members as a valuable source of information essential to understand the patient.

18. Check documents prepared about and for the patient using family and social history, a draft with the representative to make sure that it is correct before it being used or put on record as the accurate, whole truth.

19. Develop better communication protocols with the patient's representative consistent with the recommendations above on this topic.

20. Establish a single patient record system that all areas can access. Mental Health records should not be separate.

21. Review the practice for community Mental Health record keeping (Patient Progress Notes) and if limitations are

necessary, make these explicit so that professionals know what is reliable and what might be incomplete.

22. Review the transfer, including handover communications, of mental health patients from hospitals to the community and between community mental health units to reduce the risks currently built in to be led by the relevant Chief Psychiatrist.

23. Find a legal means of obtaining patients' records from a private professional where there is clinical need.

3. Health's interface with community

Health and Disability sectors not working together

It would seem that the health sector public institutions have not adjusted to the introduction of the NDIS. In particular health services showed a lack of ability to work with the disability sector with a lack of understanding of the private commercial nature of community disability organisations reliant on NDIS funding. This does not fully explain the examples of bad behaviour from health service personnel towards Alex's support coordinators, in ACT and Victoria. The overbearing rudeness seemed to be also based on an assumed superiority developed to try to control a patient's use of health services.

In the ACT, Health services and the disability sector had extreme difficulty in working together for Alex's attempts at discharge. Dhulwa was difficult to work with, assuming control of discharge planning but causing friction with the government disability department as well as Alex's community disability service providers. Why not work as a team instead of in a hierarchy with health deciding whether to engage with others?

It was particularly important for the health services to contribute to health objectives once in the community for complex cases such as Alex's. However, Dhulwa claimed that it could not envision Alex in the community so provided no mental health and physical health guidelines for disability support which it decried as useless anyway.

Disability support workers need health advice in order to know when to call for medical assistance, to know how to observe and assess symptoms. Support workers for Alex once left without guidance were learning to ignore persistent symptoms. The Royal Commission's report (September 2023)[24] included relevant findings about care responses at risk of delay and complacency.

The Victorian Regional Hospital spoke to Alex's Victorian support coordinator and the Support Worker Organisation roughly and rudely. It was trying to bully these supports into making /accepting arrangements for Alex which were not in Alex's best interests.

Health personnel kept referring to disability support workers as *NDIS workers* when they work for private organisations (utilising NDIS just as GPs utilise Medicare). Staff at NDIA

---

[24] We heard that they are also likely to have treatable pain ignored or overlooked and wait longer for a diagnosis than people without disability: if a person with disability suffers from something for long enough, momentum can be lost in terms of finding solutions. People become complacent and see health issues as just something that's 'part' of the person or disability.
    Royal Commission into Violence, Abuse, Neglect and Exploitation of People with Disability (September 2023). This material is referenced under a Creative Commons Attribution 4.0 International licence (www.creativecommons.org/licenses).

administering the NDIS have neither direct care nor coordination of that care.

The experiences in Alex's case to be highlighted are:

Experience	Specific incidents	Text
Belief facility is sufficient unto themselves even when it is clear they do not have relevant expertise	Dhulwa was not satisfied that Alex's disability support coordinator was looking for accommodation so tried to take over, giving up when it lost staff.	Ch 9
Failure of hospitals to work as a team with others involved with discharge e.g. wanting to take charge of discharge as if fully understanding the community options	Dhulwa made a mess of the planning and execution of a possible discharge in May 2020. This was largely by not fully participating in planning, not communicating and being directed by police in the manner of a trial visit to the accommodation.	Ch 9
However, assumed carer as fully responsible for all health requirements of patient whilst living in the community	Paying attention to both physical and residual mental health needs was a huge demand of support workers that needed health sector support	Ch 9

with no structured support		
Adopting right to admonish/speak rudely to community care disability organisations/workers	The Adult Mental Health Unit Canberra Hospital and the Victorian Regional Hospital were guilty of this lack of professionalism. My theory is that hospital administrations put pressure on the hospital social worker (usually) chosen as a spokesperson. The desperate hospital has to fix things by demonising anyone who might create a barrier even if arising from person centred thinking.	Ch 4 and Ch 12

Carer blaming

Once it was entrenched among health services that Alex's bad behaviour could not be treated clinically, it was also accepted that community care should manage him. There must be something wrong with workers, their qualifications and the disability system if Alex were not manageable in the community. However, the discussion went in circles when the health sector claimed only nurses could manage him such that he needs to be locked at a forensic health facility.

It was not only health services that criticised support workers. In Small Town the residents tried to give Alex's Support

Organisation a bad name, blaming them for Alex's bad behaviour. At no stage did the police or residents of this town ask why Alex was not getting adequate mental health care.

Alex's life was made difficult when carers were compromised as follows:

Experience	Specific incidents	Reference in text
Persisting with view that community arrangements are all that is required therefore those responsible are not doing their job	Time and again Alex's support coordinator was hounded about finding accommodation even when Alex was being rejected as too noisy, too volatile or having too particular living requirements. Meanwhile no review of the psychiatric approach was undertaken.	Ch 6, Ch 7
Claims that requests for medical help are being made because carers want to withdraw care (e.g. claims patient being dumped at the Regional Hospital)	The Regional Hospital even gave a parting shot to Alex's Support Organisation requesting it not dump him there again.	Ch 12

Claims carers are incompetent under circumstances of medical/health system failure	Dhulwa blamed carers for the failed discharge trial of May 2020. The Regional Hospital blamed Alex's carers for the disaster in Small Town.	Ch 8, Ch 13
Community too ready to blame carer (parents or workers) assuming medical treatment is adequate.	Small Town was quick to blame the Support Workers saying they were managing Alex badly.	Ch 13

Weaknesses in the execution of service objectives under the NDIS

The disability market has not been providing well for the fringe participants, the complex cases and those with behaviours of concern. Understandably, the first few years of the response to the introduction of the NDIS attracted providers seeking clients with the easiest to meet needs. Higher qualifications might be required for more specialist SIL providers. It is not surprising that some in the health sector are suspicious about discharge to just any organisation for community living.

The pop-up group residential places using suburban homes in the ACT might have targeted those with mental illness, for example, but were not suitable for those with both intellectual disability and mental illness. Those willing to try to accept Alex were thwarted of course by his untreated symptoms.

The SDA respite accommodation organisation in Western Melbourne was the subject of a complaint by me to the NDIS Quality and Safeguards Commission in 2023. Nearly two years later, the Commission informed me that my complaint has been moved to the Incidents Team. Such were my observed failings of the respite organisation that I concluded it was taking NDIS money without proper safeguards and supervision of standards. The organisation had limitations in business administration, execution of building standards and liaison with the disability sector. The accommodation was not a good place for someone on a physical decline combined with ongoing mental health care requirements.

There might be arguments for the return of some kinds of institutional or group care with varying degrees of restraint. Investigations into accommodation possibilities now should include these options where they can offer more supportive and less challenging environments. It might be beneficial to examine what other similar countries are doing.

Alex's experiences included:

Experience	Specific incidents	Reference in text
Creation of multiple service providers but	After two years (2018-2019) of searching for accommodation with	Ch 7

with limited experience in complex cases, preferring participants requiring simpler worker arrangements	Supported Independent Living and considering about thirty organisations before we tried interstate, no place was found suitable.	
Barriers to SDA development	The ACT has been limited for SDA because of its lack of land and its planning or zoning codes. An SDA developer has to be able to make the development viable financially through use of large or joined blocks for at least three dwellings. The ACT government has not planned for the necessary concessions.	Ch 5
Pop-up respite providers without staff which could work with Alex	Providers which quickly established an organisation would recruit support workers with suitable personal attributes, but without the depth of experience necessary to try taking Alex.	Ch 5
Limited development of	The NDIS Quality and Safeguards Commission	Ch 14

NDIS quality oversight agency	has not completed a response to my complaint. Recently, nearly two years since I made my complaint, the Commission notified me that it has been passed to the Incidents Team. There is no indication that the complaint will be expedited now.	
A quality behaviour specialist was difficult to engage creating stress and delays.	I found it was a provider's market. There are insufficient numbers of suitably qualified people and too many organisations which take short-cuts to churn out reports. I could not afford to accept low quality reports for the crucial processes with NDIA and for our aims of sustainable community living.	Chs 6, 7, 8, 9

Lack of housing in the ACT for the vulnerable

There had been much written and exposed about what is being called Australia's 'housing crisis'. The history in the ACT of public housing has been full of frustrations and sad stories for decades. I recommend reading the submission of Dr Emma

Campbell of ACTCOSS to the Inquiry by the Committee on Economy and Gender and Economic Equality into Housing and Rental Affordability 8 August 2022. Found at https://actcoss.org.au/publication/submission-inquiry-into-housing-and-rental-affordability/

My experiences with Housing ACT left me thinking that it operates under such reduced resources, its staff seek to reject applicants as much as possible. Staff adopt defensive positions precluding rational conversations and timely communications.

I noted above that the ACT government has been slow to facilitate SDA development for robust standard dwellings. A bigger effort is needed to find suitable land with associated appropriate planning rules.

Experience	Specific incidents	Text
Variable participation and communication by Housing ACT in cross-agency efforts	Housing ACT began well with the inauguration of the Multi-Agency Task Force in late 2018. They produced the letter stating Alex could get public housing and send a representative to the early meetings. Once Alex was at Dhulwa, Housing's participation deteriorated. Then it dropped its bombshell rejection in 2021.	Chs 4, 5, 6, 9

Lack of transparency in decision making by Housing ACT	For two years Housing ACT left us with the impression it was looking for accommodation for Alex.	Ch 9
Use of disabilities affecting independence to disqualify even if supported	After the period of lack of communication and updates, Housing ACT's rationale for rejecting Alex included that he was not capable of independent living and it was concerned about "ACT Housing's ability to engage and support Alex, and in turn the potential concerns regarding staff safety". This is an invented excuse. Why wouldn't any Housing administration contact be through Alex's representative and SIL organisation? Why would housing providers be expected to have the qualifications to engage directly with Alex?	Ch 9
Nonetheless interested in gaining benefits should Alex receive SDA funding.	It was not explicit but Housing showed interest in the SDA scheme and Alex's application for SDA.	Ch 10

405

Recommendations

All the recommendations above related to the potential for diagnostic overshadowing and/or mismanagement apply here in that any diagnostic and treatment failures are relayed to other health staff, affecting their willingness to blame representatives and disability carers.

24. Improve the way the health sector works with the disability sector. There should be a review of the system clashes covering the pressure to cost shift, the mostly public nature of health facilities versus the private nature of disability suppliers, poor awareness that disability workers are not community nurses and additional measures might be required for mental and physical health access, and understanding of the role of restraint and restrictive practices.

25. Educate the health sector about the disability care system! Whose responsibility is this? NDIA as the new partner in the system could reach out to the Health Departments.

26. Health administrators to inwardly review so that Health facilities are clearer about what they see as their roles as complementary to community personnel but also be prepared to work across the inside/outside frame with the community team.

27. Develop protocols for seeking independent external advice to supplement shortcomings in qualifications and experience when the wide range of patients potentially

under care in a facility is not covered, particularly if their own resources are curtailed.

28. Build a patient-centred understanding from all available information, avoiding pride which could prevent seeking help from others. Different facilities within a jurisdiction's mental health system should not see themselves as in competition.

29. Develop protocols within the health sector covering client health status observations and health management by disability carers.

30. Properly fund the NDIS Quality and Safeguards Commission.

31. Review State and Territory planning laws affecting SDA and take a proactive approach to making SDA happen and in areas with access to services required by those with disabilities.

32. Housing should publish its policies and approach for the vulnerable members of the public requiring housing.

33. Reconsider zoning in urban areas for revision where it currently prevents development of SDA.

34. Undertake allocation of areas for housing for the vulnerable just as areas are set aside for schools and community services in town planning.

The remainder of what needs to be addressed is part of a huge national housing problem in general.

Epilogue

We held a memorial service for Alex in Canberra in April 2023. I wanted the service to present Alex as far more than his last five years as a frightening misfit. I wanted his love for all of us to shine in his story. Alex's father had a serious fall on his return to Canberra after Alex died, breaking his femur, but was able to attend the service in a wheelchair. Ewen spoke about Alex as a good caring brother. We gave a biography in slides from babyhood to his trip to the theatre in February. Carers, including Serena and his Canberran carers, spoke of their love for Alex and his value as a person, including one worker singing a pertinent song of his own composition accompanied by his guitar. We displayed mementos of all Alex's activities in sport, drama and photography. We also gave a slide show of Alex's art accompanied by *Starry, Starry Night* by Don Maclean.

This song is about Vincent van Gogh (1853-1890) and the parallels with Alex are obvious: untreated illness, art and early death. The lyrics cover many of Vincent's subjects for his paintings. Clive set up the slide show so that Alex's paintings of the similar subjects appeared in time with the lyrics. Alex particularly liked Vincent Van Gogh's pictures. The only framed print he owned was a Van Gogh landscape. The only art book he bought solely on one artist was about Van Gogh. Despite Alex's art being naïve his pieces are still striking and I have kept them.

Vincent suffered from bipolar disorder and his inspired prolific painting was accomplished in his phases of mania. Of course, in his time in the nineteenth century there was no understanding of this disorder and no treatment anyway. Vincent was able to have respite rather than treatment in French mental hospitals but the closest diagnosis of any of the doctors was "epilepsy". The lyrics of the song also emphasise how Vincent was not understood by those around him. The song ends with "perhaps they never will" evoking the tragedy of it all.

Vincent had found relationships difficult and suffered many people turning away from him. Vincent was very intelligent and knew he was mentally ill. He kept trying to find his own way of coping. Art was a huge source of relief when it calmed him down as it did when he painted what was directly in front of him, rather than from imagination. His brother Theo supported him to be able to keep painting which did not bring in an income until after his death. Vincent could be posthumously diagnosed from his detailed, almost daily, accounts of his thoughts and activities to Theo and from other reports.

In the period leading up to his intense crises and eventual suicide, Vincent stayed several months in Arles in southern France in 1888. He was brought to police notice with residents fearful. While he was in hospital after a crisis there (in which he sliced his own ear) the people of Arles sent a petition to the mayor to stop Vincent returning because, while he had not hurt anyone, he was too frightening with his disinhibition, loudness and rambling, persistent talk[25]

Alex was also misunderstood and felt desperately lonely at times and he suffered from a lack of proper diagnosis about his mania. In the twenty-first century there is still ignorance among psychiatrists. Without a proper diagnosis the treatment could not be appropriate, even though we are more advanced with available treatments than in Vincent's time. Alex's cognitive disabilities worked against him getting proper mental health care. It fostered discrimination against him for access to care. He was not able to tell people about his thinking according to psychiatrists' standard formulaic questions and while the mental health system sees a benefit in trying to shift responsibility to another sector.

Alex suffered from the reactions of the people of Small Town, who wrote a petition to try to prevent him living there. The local police wanted him gone. At least the more-kindly people of Arles did not threaten to physically assault Vincent as some people of Small Town threatened to do to Alex. Ignorance of mental illness has not improved much since the nineteenth century despite improvements in education. Perhaps in the twenty-first century, people assume that all mental illness is treatable and treated, so anyone behaving in public as Alex was perceived to behave, is regarded as just evil.

Alex has the occupation of "artist" on his death certificate.

---

[25] Chapter 12 *Aftermath* in The Yellow House: Van Gogh, Gaughan and Nine Turbulent Weeks in Arles by Martin Gayford, Penguin Books 2007

I wrote to the Small Town police after Alex died to ask them to pass on the message to the family of the young boy Alex scared, that when Alex was on better medication, he said he was sorry for what he did. I received no reply, no confirmation that the police did this.

In Victoria there is a legal obligation to have a coronial inquiry for someone dying whilst in care. The coroner's scope under these circumstances is necessarily narrow and only covered treatment and events proximal to Alex's death. The report is now published with no findings warranting any recommendations for improvement in that domain.

The contact I had from ACT Health while he was dying was about the release of his confidential information among others by nurses at Dhulwa which has been in the Canberra news but I was in ignorance while in Victoria. Personal health records of several clients were involved. I was able to cope with a meeting with ACT Health on returning to Canberra and was of course horrified. I feel pain for Alex treated as a non-person, for the potential for misinterpretation of whatever information was released and for further misjudgements about him by ignorant members of the public. The action the nurses took was morally and professionally wrong. They ignored the patients' rights. They forgot them as human beings.

The rationale from the nurses for the unprofessional breaches was about their belief that management was not doing anything about the nurses' safety while undertaking their duties. I do not know anything about the other clients, but I do know that Alex was very ill, in full blown psychosis at the time of most concern by the nurses early 2022. It was the period immediately after his life-threatening illness when his antipsychotic medication had to be removed to save his life. It seems that their system catered (somewhat) for patients being at least partially treated but not for patients with florid symptoms.

It was disappointing that Alex's nurses were not handling the situation and felt at risk. I am told improvements have been introduced into Dhulwa since the 2022 review so there is optimism that the environmental problems Alex experienced will not prevail. Mental health nurses should have greater awareness of the manifestations of mental illness as a start. Dhulwa management should have anticipated the extreme situation once Alex had no medication. It seems to me that the nurses at Dhulwa were taken by surprise by someone so mentally ill and Dhulwa as an institution was not prepared for such a situation.

Of course, all these challenges would have been reduced if Alex had been correctly diagnosed from the start. They never did understand him before his death.

The Victorian dual expert psychiatrist completed her report on Alex after his death. The expert confirmed that mania should have been recognised in Alex. The report noted the deteriorations on the several occasions when his medications were withdrawn, which was done for various reasons. It also noted that his changing functioning and moods could have been influenced by a progressive neurological decline due to his rare mutation about which so little is known. In summing up where the lessons from Alex's story for the health and disability systems lie, the expert wrote:

Structural and system issues include the lack of training and expertise of health professionals in assessing and diagnosing mental illness in people with disabilities, the limited allocated clinical time and discontinuities in care, limited specialist support services, poor integration of disability, health and mental health sectors, and the real-life challenges of managing multifactorial clinical complexities in overstretched under-resourced mental health services.

Diagnostic overshadowing is a well-recognised and common cognitive bias whereby behaviour changes related to medical and mental illnesses are attributed to intellectual or other disability. Alex's concerning presentations with manic symptoms, in the presence and absence of psychotic symptoms, have over the years often been attributed to intellectual disability, despite multiple risk factors for serious mental illness and documented diagnoses of schizophrenia, mania, and schizoaffective disorder. Failure to recognise, and at times outright denial, that Alex was manic, and psychotic, resulted in delays in accessing mental health services and effective treatments, and on occasions cessation of effective treatments.[26]

---

[26] S. Cooper, C. Melville, and S. Einfeld, 'Psychiatric diagnosis, intellectual disabilities and Diagnostic Criteria for Psychiatric Disorders for Use with Adults with Learning Disabilities/Mental

Alex died prematurely in these circumstances of poorly targeted treatment of mental illness, severe restrictions on normal living and disregard for physical health, concomitant with lack of appropriate psychiatric oversight to reduce the risk of what finished him, an adverse reaction to his medication. He was bewildered, reacting strongly about the wrongs done to him as not what life was supposed to be. The slow process of eventually killing him over five years meant he lived in misery with feelings of being tortured all the while.

Will anyone listen now?

Retardation(DC-LD)' (2003) 47(1) *Journal* of *Intellectual Disability Research 3-15*

Attachment - ASH1L de novo mutation

Alex's fundamental diagnosis

There had been several suggestions from consultant psychiatrists over the years that a genetic basis for Alex's complex presentation should be explored. In 2009 a normal chromosome spread had been found. There had been confusion over whether the genetic testing was for depression or broad disabilities. Most doctors had been thinking about inherited genes, particularly thinking about what mental illness, highlighting depression, had been in the family. Alex as a whole was not like any known family member on either side so inherited genes were not uppermost in my mind. The matter was not pursued while Alex was doing well.

With Alex's admission to the Adult Mental Health Unit in 2017 and an insistence that he had behavioural problems plus mental illness, genetic studies were again suggested. Whole exome sequencing was performed in 2019 for Alex, and both parents, following a negative finding for Fragile X. The reporting of the analysis was delayed until September 2020 for various reasons, including the COVID pandemic.

A heterozygous variant designated as pathogenic in the ASH1L gene c.4039-4043delAAAAA [p. (Lys1347Glufz*7)] was identified for Alex (Canberra Clinical Genomics, ACT Genetics Service, 2020). This mutation was a *de novo* variant not present in either parent. It was a frameshift small deletion in exon 3 of 28 predicted to be responsible for loss of function as an autosomal dominant mutation. The diagnosis was confirmed by Sanger sequencing. This variant is not present in ClinVar or other public databases. Multiple other ASH1L mutations are reported in ClinVar (2023). The finding of this variant in Alex comprised the first and only explanation for his intellectual disabilities and autistic symptoms and linkage to increased risk for his comorbidities, that is for his collective neurological problems.

Gene variations at ASH1L on chromosome 1q22 have had increased attention (OMIM Clinical Synopsis #617796) associated with neurodevelopmental disorders. The published data include phenotypic descriptions in children but with nothing on the consequent adult characteristics. ASH1L encodes histone methyltransferases suggesting a major role in modulation of neuronal connectivity. Cheon et al. (2020) reported that ASH1L regulates neuronal morphogenesis by counteracting the catalytic activity of Polycomb Repressive complex 2 group (PRC2) in stem cell-derived human neurons. They concluded that ASH1L epigenetically regulates neuronal connectivity by modulating the (Trithorax group) BDNF-TrkB signalling pathway, which likely contributes to neurodevelopmental pathogenesis. This is far from any science I have ever studied but I have expressed it as well as I can from the papers.

The OMIM Clinical synopsis outlines the evidence that autosomal dominant "mental retardation"- 52 is caused by heterozygous mutation in ASH1L on chromosome 1q22. ASH1L mutations give rise to heterogeneic phenotypes, possibly because of variations in type of mutation and the complexity of the many steps from gene expression to physiology and the multiple other neurodevelopment genes requiring ASH1L proper functioning. The downstream molecular targets of the overall genes being expressed in the regulation of synaptic tissue, neuron projection, and axon growth mean that ASH1L dysfunction can affect stages from selection of neural progenitor cells to terminal dendritic differentiation and connectivity of neurons and synaptic development.

Mutations in gene ASH1L have been reported to be linked to intellectual disability (Okamoto et al., 2017), autism (Wang et al., 2016), Tourette's syndrome (Liu et al., 2019), and epilepsy (Stessman et al., 2017, Chow et al., 2019 and Tang et al., 2020). Zhang et al. (2020) noted heterozygous mutations at ASH1L are strongly enriched for variants likely to increase the risk for neurological disorders including Attention Deficit Disorder and Multiple Congenital Malformation with intellectual disability and schizophrenia, citing multiple studies. For further information on the available data supporting an association between ASH1L variants and schizophrenia, see Schizophrenia Exome Sequencing Meta-Analysis (SCHEMA) bowser (https://schema.broadinstitute.org/gene/ENSG00000116539).

The earliest reports of neurodevelopmental disorders associated with ASH1L found missense mutations which were associated with severe intellectual disability (de Ligt et al., 2012; Wang et al., 2016; Okamoto et al., 2017). In distinction, and consistent with the diagnosis of mild intellectual disability for Alex who had a frameshift mutation, Shen et al. (2019), reported a *de novo*, frameshift variant of ASH1L thought to be responsible for a patient's mild intellectual disability and multiple congenital abnormalities. The authors refer to an "emergent neurodevelopmental disorder" linked to various mutations at ASH1L. They recognised that the gene dysfunction could manifest in more than one disorder. Each case they checked was different. Their own case was different from Alex but common features were fine motor developmental delay, learning difficulties, and perhaps, sleep apnoea. They noted a broad spectrum of clinical facial features and feeding disorders may be associated with the mutations.

Zhang et al. (2020) reviewed the literature on ASH1L, having started with an interest in the role of this gene in the development of Tourette's syndrome. Tourette's syndrome has genetic inheritable properties but no single gene has been found directly responsible, so they queried the genetic basis. The authors suggest overlapping mechanisms are responsible for differently recognised neuropathologies of each of Tourette's, autism spectrum disorder, attention deficit disorder and schizophrenia. Connectivity abnormalities, neuronal circuit problems, brain networks and excitatory/inhibitory imbalance are core parts of the pathology of these diseases. It is not that a single gene mutation would be found solely responsible for the range of diseases, but aspects of abnormal gene expression can converge in the common biochemical pathways involved, perhaps originating from loss of ASH1L function.

It is possible that the findings in those with de novo mutations without family clusters of the traits indicates that the mutation conveys poor fecundity. That is, those affected do not have children.

There have been studies in mice with an introduced homozygous inability to have a normal ASH1L function. Goa et al. (2021) reported that loss of ASH1L function in the developing mouse brain alone is sufficient to cause multiple developmental defects, core autistic behaviours and impaired cognitive memory. In addition to links to autism and intellectual disability, this report notes hypothalamus dysfunctions that affect normal feeding behaviours and postnatal growth including craniofacial deformities. This is of interest when reflecting on Alex's post-natal feeding problems and the jaw growth for which he had corrective surgery later. These authors undertook gene expression analysis in neuroprogenitor cells and suggest that impaired expression of neurodevelopment genes is likely to be a main molecular mechanism linking ASH1L mutations to abnormal brain development.

More research is required to uncover the mechanisms for loss of function of ASH1L to cause each individual cluster of syndromes and diseases. From understanding those mechanisms, better medication can be developed and better pharmacological regimes can be devised. It might be that the developing field of pharmacogenomics can be applied to cases such as Alex in which responses to medication can be predicted based on their genes.

ASH1L is implicated in more than one system and one disease aetiology. Its predominant role seems to be in the brain and nervous system.

References on the ASH1L mutation

Cheon, S.H., Culver A.M., Bagnell, A.M., Ritchie, F.D., Clytus, J.M., McCord, M., Papendorp, C. M., Chukwurah, E., Smith, A.J., Cowen M.H., Ghate, P.S., Davis, S.W., Liu J.S., Lizarraga, S.B. (bioRxiv Preprint 2020) ASH1L regulates the structural development of neuronal circuitry by modulating BDNF/TrkB signalling in human neurons.
doi: https://doi.org/10.1101/2020.02.18.954586.

Chow, J., Jensen. M., Amini, H., Hormozdiari, F., Penn, O., Shifman, S., Girirajan, S. and Hormozdiari, F. (2019) Dissecting the genetic basis of comorbid epilepsy phenotypes in neurodevelopmental disorders. *Genome Medicine 11*, 65

de Ligt, J. Willemsen. M.H., van Bon, B.W.M., Kleefstra, T., Yntema, H.G., Kroes, T., Vulto-van Silfhout, A.T., Koolen, D.A., de Vries, P., Gilssen. C., del Rosario, M., Vissers, L.E.L.M. (2012) Diagnostic exome sequencing in persons with severe intellectual disability. *New England Journal of Medicine 367*, 1921-1929.

Goa, Y., Duque-Wilckens, N., Aljazi M.B., Wu Y., Moeser A.J., Mias, G.I., Robison, A.J. and He, J (2021) Loss of histone methyltransferase ASH1L in the developing mouse brain causes autistic-like behaviours *Nature Communications Biology* 4:756. doi.org/10.1038/s42003-021-12282-z.

Liu, S., Tian, M., He, F., Li, J., Xie, H. Liu, W., Zhang, Y., Zhang, R., Yi, M., Che, F., Ma, X., Zheng, Y., Deng, H., Wang, G., Chen, L., Sun, X., Xu, Y., Wang, J., Zang, Y., Han, M., and 28 others (2020) Mutations in ASH1L confer susceptibility to Tourette syndrome. *Molecular Psychiatry*, 25(2), 476-490.

Okamoto, N., Miya, F., Tsunoda T., Kato, M., Saitoh, S., Yamasaki, M., Kanemura, Y. and Kosaki K. (2017) Novel MCA/ID syndrome with ASH1L mutation. *American Journal of Medical Genetics, 173A*, 1644-1648.

OMIM clinical synopsis entry for MCD52:
http://www.omim.org/clinicalSynopsis/617796.

SCHEMA bowser
https://schema.broadinstitute.org/gene/ENSG00000116539

Shen, W., P., Rutz, A.M., Bayrak-Toydemir, P. and Dugan SL (2019) *De novo* loss-of-function variants of ASH1L are associated with an emergent neurodevelopmental disorder. *European Journal of Medical Genetics, 62*, 55-60.

Stessman, H.A.F., Xiong, B., Coe, B.P., Wang. T., Hoekzema, K., Fenckova, Kvarnung, M., Gerdts, J., Trinh, S., Cosemans, N., Vives, L., Lin, J., Turner, T.N., Santen, G., Ruivenkamp, C., Kriek, M., van Haeringen, A., Aten, E., Friend, K., Jan Liebelt, J., ...Eichler, E. E. (2017) Targeted sequencing identifies 91 neurodevelopmental-disorder risk genes with autism and developmental-disability biases. *Nature Genetics*, 49, 515-526.

Tang, S., Addis, L., Smith, A., Topp, S.T., Pendziwiat, M., Mei, D., Parker A., Agrawal, S., Hughes, E., Lascelles, K., Williams, R.E., Fallon, P., Robinson, R., Cross, H.J., Hedderly, T., Eltze, C., Kerr, T., Desurkar, A., Hussain, N., Kinali, M., ...Pal, D.K. (2020) Phenotypic and genetic spectrum of epilepsy with myoclonic atonic seizures. Epilepsia, 61(5), 995-1007.

Wang, T., Guo, H., Xiong, B., Stessman. H.A.F., Wu, H., Coe. B., Turner, T.N., Liu. L., Zhao. W., Hoekzema, K., Vivis, L., Xia, L., Tang, M., Ou. J., Chen. B., Shen Y., Xun, G., Long, M., Lin, J., Kronenberg, Z.N.,......Eichler, E.E. (2016) De novo genetic mutations among a Chinese autism spectrum disorder cohort. Nature Communications, 7: 13316. Electronic article: doi: 10.1038/ncomms13316 (2016).

Zhang, C., Xu, L., Zheng, X., Liu, S., Che, F. (2020) Role of ASH1L in Tourette syndrome and other neurodevelopmental disorders. *Developmental Neurobiology* doi: 10.1002/dneu.22795. (March, 2021) *Developmental Neurobiology 81(2)*. 79-91.

www.ingramcontent.com/pod-product-compliance
Lightning Source LLC
Chambersburg PA
CBHW051522020426
42333CB00016B/1744

"Sensing his students' loss of identity within a disenchanted world, Ray Robles offers the genuine antidote of stability found within ancient faith. The result is a much-needed book that turns to the Great Tradition of the church to make sense of the story of the Scriptures. Robles is rightly critical of early modern philosophical choices that have led to the fragmentation of being and the celebration of power. *The Ancient Story of God-With-Us* explains why we should avoid pitting Spirit over against tradition by offering a Spirit-guided return to the ancient faith. Readable yet well-informed, this book recalls why God is closer to us than we are to ourselves."
—HANS BOERSMA,
Saint Benedict Servants of Christ Chair in Ascetical Theology,
Nashotah House Theological Seminary

"The reader uninitiated with the history and thought the church awaits a wild ride through Robles's account of the activity of the triune God. Robles's explanation and exhortation arise from questions and issues students and congregants bring to him which reveal deep deficiencies in their foundational understanding of the God who is with us."
—SEAN MCGEVER,
adjunct faculty, Grand Canyon University

"Ray Robles' *The Ancient Story of God-With-Us* is a timely call for the church to rediscover its roots while remaining attuned to the Spirit's movement today. Years ago, Ray and I met at a moment when I was frustrated with the direction many churches seemed to be heading. His gentle yet piercing admonition—'You're not kicking far back enough'—stirred something in me that I didn't know I needed. This book invites readers to do the same: to kick back into the deep well of our ancient faith and, in the process, rediscover who we are. Ray's wisdom and conviction shine on every page, offering a fresh yet timeless vision for the church's future."
—D. A. SHERRON,
senior pastor, Global Fire Church

"By recovering Christian theology's proper subject matter—the nature, identity, and purposes of the triune God—Ray Robles offers much needed ballast to Christians who are anxious about the future. A timely book!"
—**JASON E. VICKERS**,
William J. Abraham Professor of Theology and Wesleyan Studies, Baylor University, Truett Seminary